Personalizing Health Action Plans
A Student Resource Manual

for

Pruitt and Stein
HealthStyles
Decisions for Living Well

Second Edition

prepared by

John L. Rohwer
Bethel College

Robert Wandberg
Bethel College

Allyn and Bacon
Boston London Toronto Sydney Tokyo Singapore

TABLE OF CONTENTS

1   Health: Your Personal Responsibility 1

2   Assessing Your Health: A Plan for Informed Decision-making 9

3   Managing Your Mental Health 19

4   Coping With Stress 29

5   Eating Smart 37

6   Maintaining Proper Weight 45

7   Keeping Fit 55

8   Smoking Out Tobacco 63

9   Dealing With Drinking 73

10 Understanding the Dangers of Drug Use 83

11 Recognizing Violent Behavior 93

12 Preventing Unntentional Injuries 103

13 Reducing the Risk of Chronic Disease 113

14 Reducing the Risk of Infectious Disease 123

15 Reducing the Risk of Sexually Transmitted Diseases 133

16 Sexuality: Developing Healthy Relationships 143

SPECIAL: Your Sexual Body: A Primer on Reproductive Anatomy and Physiology 153

17 Planning a Family 159

18 Aging: Growing Older, Keeping Healthy 169

19 Death and Dying 179

20 Living in a Healthy Environment 189

21 Making Health Care Decisions 199

PREFACE TO THE STUDENT RESOURCE MANUAL

This Student Resource Manual has been developed to complement Healthstyles: Decisions for Living Well by Pruitt and Stein. Each chapter in the Manual includes elements designed to enable you, the learner, not only to remember the facts, but also an opportunity to develop the curiosity and mental discipline necessary to pursue answers to questions.

This manual is divided into five major sections: Chapter Overview, Chapter Focus Questions, Case Study Reflections, Chapter Activities, and Chapter Review Test. The following is an explanation of each section as they correspond with each chapter in the Healthstyles: Decisions for Living Well textbook:

Chapter Overview
The chapter overview provides a brief, yet comprehensive, description of the major concepts found in that chapter.

Chapter Focus Questions
Ten learning objectives provide an awareness of the information, both factual and conceptual, to be learned from each chapter. After reading each chapter you should be able to answer each question.

Case Study Reflections
Questions from the textbook case studies have been generated to assist you in the area of critical thinking analysis. The questions enable you to visualize the possible, likely, and essential consequences of different beliefs and actions; explain the perspective of others; challenge one's own and others' assumptions; all of which enhance critical thinking.

Chapter Activities
Each chapter has three distinct chapter activities to assist you in deepening your learning and understanding of the chapter content: (1) A Personal Assessment section — designed to assist you in determining a personal connection and relevance to the chapter content; (2) A Health Enhancement section — designed to extend and enrich your learning; and (3) A Health Promotion section — designed to assist you in determining ways you could be a health advocate for your family, friends, and community.

Chapter Review Test
The practice or review test follows the student activities section in each chapter. Use the test to check your retention of information. Following each test question is the corresponding page number where the material for that question can be located in the chapter. In addition, the key (answer section) for each chapter test is located in the back of the Resource Manual.

CHAPTER 1
HEALTH: YOUR PERSONAL RESPONSIBILITY

Chapter Overview

This chapter lays the framework for the rest of the textbook by explaining the meaning of health, and how important it is for an individual to develop and maintain a positive healthstyle.

Defining Health. The World Health Organization (WHO) defines health as "a state of complete physical, mental and social well-being and not merely the absence of disease or infirmity." This definition regards health as holistic; that is, engaging all aspects of an individual. The idea that an individual has potential for good health and a responsibility in living up to that potential, despite limitations or disabilities, is a concept called *wellness*.

Becoming Healthy. To become healthy, an individual can develop healthy behaviors, or change unhealthy habits. An individual's healthstyle includes three factors; *health knowledge*, *Healthskills* and *health behavior*. These determine one's health choices. To make correct choices, *health knowledge* assumes that an individual is able to acquire accurate and reliable health information, be able to effectively learn from the information and is willing to relay this information for the benefit of others. Good *Healthskills* are of assistance in day-to-day living, working, leisure, and in the ability to learn. They include motor skills, intellectual skills, emotional skills, and social skills. *Health behaviors,* the actions people employ when confronted with health issues, include *preventive behavior, illness behavior* or the actions taken when someone experiences certain symptoms, and *sick-role behavior* or the way a person will take care of themselves once diagnosed with an illness.

Establishing a Personal Healthstyle. In addition to health behaviors, skills, and knowledge, healthstyle includes health values, attitudes, beliefs, culture, and environment. A third component to healthstyle is called the *health momentum*, or the likelihood that once a healthy or unhealthy action is taken it will be repeated.

Prevention: The Best Alternative. Most causes of death in this country are the result of a disease that has been caused or aggravated by unhealthy behaviors. The best way to protect against disease is through prevention. Prevention includes obtaining facts and making healthy choices based on accurate information and common sense. Once a healthy decision is made, then actions can be taken to modify behavior. For example, not smoking, regular exercise, nutritious diet, controlled alcohol consumption, and practicing safer sex will all reduce one's risk of disease and lead to a better quality of life. The responsible individual who is concerned about his/her health will practice common sense, use learned Healthskills and engage in constructive and healthy behavior.

There are three **Critical Thinking Questions** throughout the text. The first discusses the lack of preventative assistance given patients by the medical profession; the second questions whether or not wearing motor cycle helmets is an issue of public health policy; and the third examines diseases that can only be 'cured' with prevention.

Chapter Focus Questions

1.   How would you describe a healthy person?

2.   What is involved in the process of becoming healthy?

3.   How is health knowledge related to your overall well-being?

4.   How are health skills related to your overall well-being?

5.   How is healthy development different from health behavior change?

6.   What are the factors that influence components of a healthy lifestyle?

7.   How do health beliefs and health attitudes influence health style?

8.   How do personal health decisions create a health momentum?

9.   What is meant by prevention education and how does it apply to life?

10.   Why is it said that good health practices often come down to common sense?

Case Study Reflections

Chapter one begins with a focus on the values one places on his/her health. Maria places a high value on health and actively maintains physical well-being. Phil, on the other hand, regards health less seriously and takes a passive approach to his physical fitness.

1. What reason(s) account for Maria's success at practicing a healthy lifestyle?

2. What accounts for Phil's failure at practicing a healthy lifestyle?

3. Imagine that Phil is a friend of yours. One day you hear him bragging about his unhealthy lifestyle. How would you respond? Is there anything you could say to change his attitude? If so, what?

4. Later, Phil tells you that he desires a more healthy lifestyle. What three suggestions for change of behavior would you make? Why?

Chapter Activities

A.   Personal Assessment:
Am I "health literate?" To find out, circle the answer that best applies to you.

	Never		Sometimes		Always
1. I am a critical thinker and problem solver who is able to identify and creatively address health problems and issues at multiple levels ranging from personal to international.	1	2	3	4	5
2. I am able to utilize a variety of resources to access the current, credible and application information required to make sound health-related decisions.	1	2	3	4	5
3. I am a responsible productive citizen who realizes my obligation to ensure that my community is kept healthy, safe, and secure.	1	2	3	4	5
4. I avoid behaviors which pose a health or safety threat to myself or others.	1	2	3	4	5
5. I am a self-directed learner who has command of the dynamic health promotion and disease prevention knowledge base.	1	2	3	4	5
6. I can apply healthy interpersonal and social skills in relationships.	1	2	3	4	5
7. I can effectively communicate beliefs, ideas and information about health.	1	2	3	4	5
8. I advocate for positions, policies, and programs that are in the best interest of society and intended to enhance personal, family, and community health.	1	2	3	4	5

Conclusion:

1.   Add up your score. The maximum score is 40. The higher the score, the more "health literate" you are.

2.   Which area(s) did you score the highest (4 or 5 points)?_____
_____

3.   Which area(s) did you score the lowest (1 or 2 points)?_____

_____

4.   What is one change I could make to improve my health literacy?_____

_____

B.   Health Enhancement:

1.   Using the personal health literacy assessment, interview several family members and/or friends to determine their health literacy. Prepare a chart or graph to summarize your findings.
2.   Create a design and slogan for a bumper sticker that encourages improved health literacy. Share your bumper sticker with the class.
3.   Interview an older person. Ask how the health issues or problems of today are similar or different from years ago.

C.   Health Promotion:

1.   List three ways you could be involved in improving the health literacy of the general population.
2.   List three ways cultural, environmental (physical or social-economic), political, religious, or health care attitudes/actions could be directly or indirectly involved in improving the health literacy of the general population.
3.   Suggest one way that you personally could be a "health literacy" advocate for each of the two target groups: (1) family; (2) friends.

Chapter Review Test

Multiple Choice: Directions: In the space at the left, write the letter of the choice that best completes each of the following statements:

_____   1. The concept of wellness is (p. 4)
   a. the achievement of total physical fitness
   b. holistic health
   c. one's potential and responsibility for health
   d. the ability to adapt successfully

_____   2. According to Halbert Dunn, an individual's level of wellness depends on (pp. 4-5)
   a. the total individual
   b. direction and progress
   c. how the individual functions
   d. all of the above

_____   3. The process of becoming healthy is most influenced by which combination of factors? (pp.5-6)
   a. knowledge, skills and behaviors
   b. parents, friends and community
   c. resources, facilities and opportunity
   d. culture, religion and politics

_____   4. According to the National Health Education Standards, health literacy means (p.7)
   a. adjusting to changes and challenges in a rapidly changing world
   b. ways of communicating with others
   c. lifestyle choices
   d. interpreting, understanding and using basic health information in ways that enhance the health of self and others

_____   5. The information that is needed to develop health literacy, maintain and improve health, prevent disease, and reduce health-related behaviors is/are referred to as: (p.6)
   a. health knowledge
   b. resistance skills
   c. health skills
   d. resiliency factors

_____   6. Actions that promote health literacy, maintain and improve health, prevent disease and reduce health-related risk behavior are: (p.8)
   a. protective factors
   b. health skills
   c. resistance skills
   d. resiliency factors

_____ 7. A set of actions and reactions to a variety of stimuli which may lead to enhancing and protecting one's health status or to its decline is called: (p.10)
  a. an attitude
  b. health behavior
  c. a belief
  d. a cue to action

_____ 8. A heroin addict given methadone through a local treatment program is an example of. (p.11)
  a. wellness behavior
  b. sick-role behavior
  c. illness behavior
  d. preventive behavior

_____ 9. Getting immunized against diseases such as polio is an example of: (p.10)
  a. preventive behavior
  b. illness behavior
  c. sick-role behavior
  d. health promotion

_____ 10. Attending a smoking cessation program in an effort to quit the habit of smoking is an example of: (p. 11)
  a. preventive behavior
  b. illness behavior
  c. sick-role behavior
  d. health promotion

_____ 11. A person's health style (lifestyle) is influenced by one's attitudes, beliefs, values and (p.13)
  a. health momentum
  b. well-being
  c. intellect
  d. emotions

_____ 12. Reducing the likelihood of smoking by exercising regularly is an example of: (p.13)
  a. health momentum
  b. homeostasis
  c. intellectualizing
  d. emotional stability

_____ 13. Today, most of the leading causes of illness and death result from: (p.14)
  a. one's genetic make-up
  b. the availability of health care services
  c. the environment
  d. one's health compromising behaviors

_____   14. The two most rapidly growing actual causes of death in this country are: (p.14)
      a. heart disease and cancer
      b. sexual behavior and drug use
      c. pneumonia and influenza
      d. AIDS and stroke

_____   15. Taking steps that stop a health problem before it starts is called: (p.15)
      a. wellness
      b. health promotion
      c. prevention
      d. prevalence

CHAPTER 2
ASSESSING YOUR HEALTH: A PLAN FOR INFORMED DECISION-MAKING

Chapter Overview

Good health practices can be taught, but it is up to the individual to take action to live a healthy life. This chapter discusses the individual's responsibility towards health, concentrating on reducing one's own health risks and how to recognize, monitor and define those health risks.

Why a Health Assessment? A health assessment provides *baseline data* which helps to make correct decisions regarding one's health. A *primary health assessment* is used to determine a person's state of health with no known disease or illness present, while a *secondary health assessment* is used for diagnosis and treatment of existing health problems. Some of the problems that occur with health assessments are laboratory inaccuracies and patients' erroneous reports of their state of health or their health-related behaviors. *Epidemiologists* study epidemics, which are diseases affecting a given population, studying *incidence data* which counts the total number of cases, *morbidity data* and *life expectancy* rates. When a disease is constant within a community, it is considered *endemic*. When the disease affects most of the world, it is *pandemic*.

National Goals for the Year 2000. The U.S. Public Health Service established a national health assessment process, called *Healthy People 2000* which instituted specific health goals for all Americans that are desired by the year 2000. These goals are to: (1) increase the life span of Americans, (2) decrease health disparities among different groups of Americans, and (3) provide accessible prevention services for all Americans. Twenty-two health issues (for example: Nutrition, Environmental Health and Cancer) are grouped under three categories called *health promotion, health protection*, and *preventive services*. This textbook is organized to examine each of the 22 health issues.

Assessing Your Personal Health. When a *health risk assessment* is undertaken by an individual in conjunction with a trained physician, potential *risk factors* are determined. It is after the risk factors have been identified that suggestions are made to modify behaviors and/or the surrounding environment to reduce the chances of disease. One such assessment is a *health risk appraisal*. An appraisal uses any variety of methods which determine the probability an individual has for acquiring a specific type of disease. One example is a self-questionnaire to determine personal health habits. One is included in this chapter. Theorists throughout the twentieth century have proposed strategies for changing health behaviors. If change is to be successful two things are necessary: individuals must take some personal responsibility in improving their behavior and actually desire a change.

Healthskills: Assessing, Recording, Changing. Collecting your own health data and updating it throughout your life is an important way to manage your health. Measuring body temperature, pulse, keeping track of changes in your weight, checking breasts or testes for signs of lumps as well as other parts of your body for any abnormalities are all ways to monitor your health. Also, a trained physician should conduct a medical assessment that includes a physical examination, an analysis of your family history and laboratory testing for any diseases. Keeping your own records of each disease, cold, illness, examination, laboratory result, prescription usage and adverse reaction to substances, will assist you in controlling and maintaining your health.

There are four **Critical Thinking Questions** interjected throughout the text. They include: (1) the subjective assessments of one's health; (2) the ethics of reporting diseases which may jeopardize people's privacy; (3) difficulties that may arise in interpreting physical standards; and (4) how best to detect breast cancer in its early stages.

Chapter Focus Questions

1.   What is the value of health assessments to an overall healthy lifestyle?

2.   How is health risk defined and why are some risks controllable while others are not?

3.   What is a wellness inventory and how do you describe its usefulness?

4.   What is the difference between risk age and achievable age?

5.   What are some of the problems associated with laboratory tests, particularly the occurrence of false negatives and false positives?

6.   What is a definition of epidemiology and what impact does it have on personal and community health?

7.   How does morbidity differ from mortality data?

8.   How would you describe yourself in relation to your health status?

9.   What is the value of keeping accurate, up-to-date health records?

10.   Might healthy behaviors lead to health risk reduction?

Case Study Reflections

In the beginning of chapter 2, Joe and Bob complete health assessments of themselves. Joe's faulty assessment needs correcting by a physician. Bob, on the other hand, is able to make adjustments to his health because of an appropriate self-assessment.

1.   What is the difference between the way Joe and Bob see themselves in the mirror?

2.   After reading the chapter, besides looking in the mirror, what other means would you recommend Joe and Bob incorporate to assess their health?

3.   Bob is aware of his family's history of heart disease. There is no history of heart disease in Joe's family, however. Should Joe still be concerned about heart disease? Why? Does he need to be as concerned about being overweight as Bob? Why?

4.   Bob ignored the fact that he was gaining weight. Do you think he will listen to his doctor's warning? Why or why not? What is the connection between awareness and action?

Chapter Activities

A.   **Personal Assessment:**
Do I follow the "basic health habits" which contribute to a healthier and longer life? To find out, circle the response that applies to you.

		Never		Sometimes		Always
1.	I avoid the use of tobacco.	1	2	3	4	5
2.	I get seven hours of sleep a night.	1	2	3	4	5
3.	I eat breakfast.	1	2	3	4	5
4.	I maintain normal body weight.	1	2	3	4	5
5.	I drink alcohol in moderation, if at all.	1	2	3	4	5
6.	I get exercise on a routine basis.	1	2	3	4	5
7.	I practice safer sex.	1	2	3	4	5
8.	I wear a seat belt.	1	2	3	4	5

Conclusion:
1.   Add up your score. The maximum score is 40. The higher the score, the more "basic health habits" you follow.

2.   Which area(s) did you score the highest (4 or 5 points)?_____
_____

3.   Which area(s) did you score the lowest (1 or 2 points)?_____
_____

4.   What is one change I could make to improve my basic health habits?_____
_____

B.   Health Enhancement:

1.   Prepare a 30-second radio Public Service Announcement (PSA) encouraging listeners to improve their basic health habits. Read to class.
2.   Locate magazine/newspaper advertisements for various products that either support or oppose any of the basic health habits. Share with class.
3.   Watch a TV sitcom. Site examples of how the messages support, or do not support, basic health habits.

C.   Health Promotion:

1.   List three ways you could be involved in improving the basic health habits of the general population.
2.   List three ways cultural, environmental (physical or social-economic), political, religious, or health care attitudes/actions could be directly or indirectly involved in improving the basic health habits of the general population.
3.   Suggest one way that you personally could be a "basic health habits" advocate for each of the two target groups: (1) family; (2) friends.

Chapter Review Test

Multiple Choice: Directions: In the space at the left, write the letter of the choice that best completes each of the following statements:

_____ 1. Information collected through a health assessment provides baseline data about one's: (p. 25)
   a. illness
   b. health status
   c. attitudes
   d. beliefs

_____ 2. Glucose tolerance testing for diabetes would be an example of what kind of health assessment? (p. 25)
   a. primary
   b. secondary
   c. tertiary
   d. wellness

_____ 3. To be told you have no evidence of a disease when in fact the opposite is true is an example of what type of laboratory error? (p.26)
   a. false negative
   b. false positive
   c. true negative
   d. true positive

_____ 4. The occurrence of a disease in a given population at a greater prevalence rate than would normally be expected is referred to as . (p.27)
   a. iatrogenic
   b. endemic
   c. epidemic
   d. pandemic

_____ 5. An epidemic which spreads over several countries or continents and affects a large number of people is said to be: (p. 27)
   a. epidemic
   b. pandemic
   c. outbreak
   d. endemic

_____ 6. The number or rate of cases that exist (prevail) at a specified time is called: (p. 27)
   a. prevalence rate
   b. incidence rate
   c. proportional rate
   d. incremental rate

_____ 7. Rates used to express the incidence of disease or prevalence of disease are called: (p. 28)
   a. endemic rates
   b. pandemic rates
   c. morbidity rates
   d. mortality rates

_____ 8. The goals of Healthy People 2000 include all of the following EXCEPT: (p.29)
   a. increase the span of healthy living for Americans
   b. identify the cure for every known disease among mankind
   c. reduce health disparities among Americans
   d. achieve access to preventive services for all Americans

_____ 9. An assessment conducted by a health care professional such as a physician that focuses on diagnosing whether or not you have a certain disease is known as. (p.32)
   a. health risk assessment
   b. medical assessment
   c. self-assessment
   d. primary assessment

_____ 10. Health risks are usually defined in terms of: (p.32)
   a. behaviors and environment
   b. age, gender, and income level
   c. income level and behavior
   d. knowledge, attitudes and beliefs

_____ 11. An assessment instrument using survey questions concerning an individual's health history, life style and medical status is an example of a: (p.34)
   a. self-assessment
   b. health risk appraisal
   c. medical assessment
   d. functional assessment

_____ 12. This theoretical model explains people's behavior on the basis of consequences and reinforcement. (p.35)
   a. Human Motivation Theory
   b. Levin's Field Theory
   c. Social Cognitive Theory
   d. Behavior Modification

_____ 13. This theoretical model suggests that behaviors are practiced or reinforced when they are approved or disapproved by others. (p.35)
   a. Human Motivation Theory
   b. Theory of Reasoned Action
   c. Social Cognitive Theory
   d. Behavior Modification

_____ 14. This theoretical model claims that health behavior is influenced by a person's perceived level of susceptibility and severity to a health threat: (p.35)
a. Health Belief Model
b. Theory of Reasoned Action
c. Transtheoretical Model
d. Behavior Modification

_____ 15. A physical examination involves which of the following procedures? (p.37)
a. health appraisal, diagnosis and treatment
b. inspection, listening and touching
c. health risk appraisal, consultation and testing
d. consultation, massage and medication

CHAPTER 3
MANAGING YOUR MENTAL HEALTH

Chapter Overview

Mental health can be seen as one component of a three-part system; biological, social and psychological. Mental well-being can be understood as a continuum ranging from mental health to mental illness. This chapter deals with the mentally healthy person who works to maintain his/her mental well-being.

A Continuum of Well-Being. There are many qualities that define a person as mentally well; such as the ability to maintain a constant mood, good self-esteem, flexibility and control over emotions. People experience good self-esteem, flexibility and control over emotions. People experience numerous emotions such as anger, frustration, hostility, fear, and love. How people act in response to their emotions is another way to determine if they are mentally well-adjusted. Behavioral tendencies such as sleeping habits allow the body to function well. Sleep irregularities are considered important clues to emotional difficulties.

Who Am I? The Importance of Knowing Yourself. *Self-concept* comes from a realistic assessment of your strengths and weaknesses whereas *self-esteem* shows how well you respect and value yourself. *Self-efficacy* is the belief that you can accomplish certain tasks while *self-actualization* is the real attainment of your most lofty goals.

A Continuum of Mental Dysorganization explores Karl Menninger's theory that the degree of mental illness a person will go through when experiencing problems in life is directly linked to how much dysfunction they possess. Inserted is a diagram, *A Spectrum of Mental States,* that shows the different levels of dysfunction: nervous, neurotic, openly aggressive, psychotic, and finally self-destructive. One of the most common types of mental afflictions are neuroses; examples of neurotic behavior are anxiety and phobias. Other mental problems involve forms of depression; minor depression happening to most people at certain times and major depression which can cause severe difficulties in coping with day-to-day living over a longer period of time. The different forms of severe depression are categorized as: affective disorders which include premenstrual dysphoric disorder (PMDD), seasonal affective disorder and manic-depressive illness. Other disorders, called psychoses, are extreme mental illnesses that usually require hospitalization. One very debilitating psychotic disorder is schizophrenia.

Suicide: A Symptom of Mental Illness. It is estimated that there are over 200,000 attempts at suicide, and over 30,000 people who successfully take their own lives. Professionals who study suicide, called suicidologists, find different causes stemming from psychological, biological and sociological problems and suggest that many suicides could be prevented. The highest numbers of suicides occur among the elderly and teenagers. Most people who commit suicide do it not to inflict self-destruction, but see suicide as a way to cope with their problems. Signs that many people wanting to attempt suicide will give are: substance abuse, depression, isolation, extreme pessimism and a change in normal habits.

Getting Help for Mental Health Problems lists and describes how certain professionals, psychiatrists, psychologists, social workers and mental health counselors can assist those experiencing all types of mental problems.

Healthskills: When to Call for Help. Developing skills to assess yourself well will lead you to know when you should make a decision to seek help and allow you to judge what type of help you need. The most important skill is being able to ask for help.

There are three **Critical Thinking Questions** within the chapter. The first questions the methods used in determining the number of people who need to seek treatment for mental disorders. The second asks the reader to think of useful strategies a community can employ to reduce mental disorders and the third question poses the difficulties that prevent people from using what mental health services are available to them.

Chapter Focus Questions

1.   How would you differentiate between a mentally well and a mentally ill person?

2.   What is meant by emotional and social well-being?

3.   What role do emotions play in a healthy lifestyle and what are several normal emotions along with positive and negative ways to express them?

4.   What are the mental health benefits of sleep?

5.   How are the terms self-concept, self-esteem, self-efficacy and self-actualization defined?

6.   How are the following mental illnesses defined; anxiety, depression and schizophrenia?

7.   How would you differentiate between minor depression and major depression?

8.   What are the characteristics of an individual contemplating suicide?

9.   In what ways do the various mental health professionals address emotional problems?

10.   At what point would you call for help if you suspect that you are experiencing a mental health problem?

Case Study Reflections

In the introduction to chapter 3, Marie and Charles each face debilitating depression. Eventually, they both turn to others for help. Charles, however, waits longer before dealing with his depression.

1.   After reading the chapter, recognize the traits for depression of both Marie and Charles. What symptomatic traits for depression do each display? What might be the source for their depression?

2.   With regard to their "self-concept, self-esteem, self-efficacy and self-actualization," how do Marie and Charles perceive themselves?

3.   Account for Marie's getting help and Charles' failing to do so. What social factors could be at work to explain their respective responses?

4.   Neither Marie nor Charles understands how their depression originated. How might these "inexplicable feelings" affect their views of themselves? How does it affect their getting help?

5.   Both Marie and Charles appear very alone with their depression. Why don't they turn to their friends or family for help? Why is it important to get professional help?

Chapter Activities

A: **Personal Assessment:**
Am I a mentally well-adjusted person? To find out, circle the answer that best applies to you.

		Never		Sometimes		Always
1.	I have a positive self-image and good self-esteem.	1	2	3	4	5
2.	I experience appropriate and stable moods.	1	2	3	4	5
3.	I maintain control of my emotions.	1	2	3	4	5
4.	I have the ability to love, feel guilt and accept remorse.	1	2	3	4	5
5.	I demonstrate flexibility and adaptability in social situations.	1	2	3	4	5
6.	I acknowledge personal strengths and accept personal limitations.	1	2	3	4	5
7.	I tolerate ambiguity, and understand that conflict is normal.	1	2	3	4	5
8.	I do not distort reality, consciously or unconsciously.	1	2	3	4	5
9.	I know how to obtain reliable mental health-related information, products, and services.	1	2	3	4	5

Conclusion:

1.   Add up your score. The maximum score is 45. The higher the score, the more "mentally well-adjusted" you are.

2.   Which area(s) did you score the highest (4 or 5 points)?_____
_____

3.   Which area(s) did you score the lowest (1 or 2 points)?_____
_____

4.   What is one change I could make to improve my mental health?_____
_____

B.   Health Enhancement:

1.   Read about Abraham Maslow's hierarchy of needs. Describe, in pictures or words, how a mentally healthy person could satisfy each of the needs.
2.   Think of a person you know who demonstrates a high level of mental health. Describe several characteristics that this person demonstrates in his or her daily routine.
3.   Create a directory of mental health resources in your community. What information, products, or services do they provide and what are the costs associated with each.
4.   Examine the pros and cons of using the legal defense of "temporary insanity."

C.   Health Promotion:

1.   List three ways you could be involved in improving the mental health of the general population.
2.   List three ways cultural, environmental (physical or social-economic), political, religious, or health care attitudes/actions could be directly or indirectly involved in improving the mental health of the general population.
3.   Suggest one way that you personally could be a "mental health advocate" for each of the two target groups: (1) family; (2) friends.

Chapter Review Test

Multiple Choice: Directions: In the space at the left, write the letter of the choice that best completes each of the following statements:

_____ 1. Mental health defined implies (p.49)
- a. mental illness
- b. the ability to negotiate daily challenges
- c. a state of emotional well-being
- d. a state of physical well-being

_____ 2. Two important aspects of good mental health are represented by: (p.49)
- a. knowing how to deal with one's emotions and gaining personal insight from these experiences
- b. trusting one's own reactions and accepting one's self without becoming frustrated
- c. achieving one's potentialities and saying what one means and feels
- d. all of the above

_____ 3. Characteristics associated with a mentally well person include all BUT which of the following qualities? (p. 50)
- a. maintains control of emotions
- b. demonstrates flexibility and adaptability in social situations
- c. acknowledges personal strengths and accepts personal limitations
- d. has a poor self-image and negative self-esteem

_____ 4. The barrier(s) to mental wellness include: (p. 49)
- a. genetics
- b. physical abilities
- c. social and environmental conditions
- d. all of the above

_____ 5. Frustration is a feeling best described as one of: (p.51)
- a. unhappiness and madness
- b. disappointment
- c. hostility
- d. fear

_____ 6. A positive response to fear might be displayed by: (p.51)
- a. staying at home and sleeping excessively
- b. locating the source of one's fear and restructure one's environment to eliminate the source
- c. getting in the car and taking a long drive out in the country
- d. reading a book about what fears others are experiencing

_____   7. The process of mind-body healing when protective chemicals in the brain are released
                boosting the immune system is referred to as: (p.52)
                a. neurotransmission
                b. neurohormones
                c. psychoneuroimmunology
                d. immuno-suppression

_____   8. During REM sleep all BUT which of the following experiences/reactions take place? (p. 54)
                a. the mind is active, even hyperactive
                b. acceleration of the heart rate and blood flow to the brain
                c. erections in males and engorgement of the clitoris in females
                d. sporadic movement and jerking of the skeletal muscles

_____   9. All BUT which of the following suggestions applies to getting a better night's sleep? (p. 54)
                a. go to bed and wake up at about the same time each morning
                b. avoid eating heavy meals two hours before bedtime
                c. exercise regularly, especially in the evening prior to going to bed
                d. stay away from stimulants such as coffee, cola drinks and tea before you go to bed

_____   10. Self-concept is how we __ ourselves, whereas self-esteem is how we _____ ourselves. (pp.
                54-55)
                a. see, value
                b. value, see
                c. accept, love
                d. believe in, pursue

_____   11. Self-efficacy is a belief in _____, whereas self-actualization is related to how we seek to
                _____. (p.57)
                a. how one sees oneself, value ourselves
                b. the ability to do a specific behavior, fulfill our potential
                c. pursuing safety needs, avoid negative experiences
                d. fate or chance, rationalize behavior

_____   12. A person's belief about whether he or she can successfully engage in and execute a specific
                behavior refers to: (p.57)
                a. self-esteem
                b. self-concept
                c. self-actualization
                d. self-efficacy

_____   13. The type of depression that occurs in the winter months, when sunlight levels are low, is
                called: (p.63)
                a. manic-depression illness
                b. dysphoric disorder
                c. seasonal affective disorder
                d. dementia

_____   14. The symptoms of schizophrenia include all BUT which of the following? (p.64)
  a.   altered sense of self
  b.   emotions consistent with thoughts
  c.   disordered thinking
  d.   delusions

_____   15. All of the following are warnings of a suicide, EXCEPT: (pp. 65-66)
  a.   a sense of helplessness and hopelessness
  b.   an increased interest in classes and/or work
  c.   a preoccupation with themes of death
  d.   a plan for a radical, permanent change of scene like running away from home

CHAPTER 4
COPING WITH STRESS

Chapter Overview

This chapter explains both positive stress, *eustress* and negative stress, *distress*, how to recognize different types of stress and how best to cope with stress. Included is a self-test that rates the stressors in one's life, using both positive and negative stressors as indicators.

Defining Stress. Stress is the recognition of an external experience that brings about a *stress response*, which is the internal, biological reaction to *stressors*. Stressors are considered to be outside events or situations that can occur to a person. A person can be conscious that these events are causing stress or an awareness of them entirely. Hans Selye developed the *general adaptation syndrome (GAS)* to explain his three-stage theory of the stress response. A person first reacts to a situation with an *alarm reaction*, then *resistance*, which calms the body, and finally the person experiences an *exhaustion* stage. There are different sources of stress that are generated from four main areas of life: the physical body, the environment, the psychological state, and society. **Your Environmental Neighborhood** article, "Festive Malaise," examines the myth that most severe emotional trauma occurs during the winter holiday season.

Impact of Stress on Health. There is a clear correlation between stress and physical health. Most doctors examine a majority of their patients for stress-related illnesses. The patients' symptoms stem from both *health effects*, such as migraines, insomnia or chest pains, *behavioral effects*, like emotional outbursts and impulsive behavior, as well as *subjective effects*, such as irritability, depression and apathy. Studies are listed in the text showing how stress directly affects the body's immune system.

Stressors of Everyday Living. Students in particular, whether they be making the transition from high school to college, graduate student with families or older, returning students, face multiple stressors in their lives from the unique condition of school. Workplace stress is quite widespread, especially when employees are not able to exert much control in their particular occupation.

Healthskills for Adapting to Stress. To successfully manage stress, one needs to identify stressors and develop *coping skills*, which include changing your perception of a stressful event, better management of your time and emotions. These skills are best aided with well developed *interpersonal skills*. The **Developing Healthskills** article, "Stressed Out? Develop a Healthy Style of Talking It Out," reinforces the idea that maintaining strong personal relationships will benefit both your physical and mental health. Exercise, meditation and proper relaxation techniques are other positive ways of dealing with stress.

There are four **Critical Thinking Questions** interjected throughout the text. They explore: (1) how public health policy intervention can work to control stressful environments for the community; (2) reduce noise on worksites to alleviate stress; (3) how to increase the number of people who employ healthy methods to control stress; and (4) suggestions as to why meditation, while a proven stress reducing method, is not widely practiced.

Chapter Focus Questions

1. How is stress defined and how is it a part of your daily living?

2. What are some common stressors and what is their origin?

3. What is the difference between primary stressors and secondary stressors and what is the effect of each?

4. What is meant by the statement that stress results from a reaction to events, not the events themselves?

5. What is the difference between distress and eustress?

6. How would you describe the scientific connection between too much stress and the incidence of disease?

7. Is stress in college life any different then stress in the work environment?

8. What skills are there for coping with stress including changing the perception of stressors, managing time and managing emotion?

Case Study Reflections

George and Juan both face stress in their day-to-day college lives. George adds to that stress by responding in anger and frustration. Juan, however, effectively neutralizes the stress he faces by the way he deals with it.

1. Identify the specific stressors in George and Juan's lives. Where do they come from? (Are they internal, external, physical, mental, etc.?) On a psychological level, how does the body respond to stress?

2. "After experiencing eustress people are able to relax and enjoy a feeling of peacefulness. . ." Which of these two young men, Juan or George, is experiencing eustress? Why?

3. George is a college freshman and is undecided about a major. Juan is a junior Literature Major and wants to teach. Explain the connection between their academic pursuits and the stress each feels in his life. Does this affect the manner in which they handle their stress? Why/Why not?

4. Research shows a strong tie between stress with both physical and mental health. Why is George more susceptible to physical and/or mental disorders than Juan? What steps should George take to help insure he avoids physical and mental health risks?

Chapter Activities

A.   **Personal Assessment:**
Am I stressed out? To find out, circle the answer that best applies to you.

		Never		Sometimes		Always
1.	I currently experience biological stressors such as injuries, physical or mental illnesses, or disabilities.	1	2	3	4	5
2.	I currently experience environment stressors such as noise, air, or water pollution, natural disasters, or poverty.	1	2	3	4	5
3.	I currently experience social or life stressors such as death of a loved one, divorce, or personal relationships.	1	2	3	4	5
4.	I currently experience lifestyle or behavior stressors such as alcohol, tobacco, or other drug use, financial concerns, improper eating habits, or lack of appropriate exercise.	1	2	3	4	5
5.	I currently experience new intellectual challenges.	1	2	3	4	5
6.	I currently experience time management stressors.	1	2	3	4	5
7.	I know how to obtain reliable stress-related information, products, and services.	1	2	3	4	5

Conclusion:
1.   Add up your score. The maximum score is 35. The higher the score, the more stressors you have.

2.   Which area(s) did you score the highest (4 or 5 points)?_____
_____

3.   Which area(s) did you score the lowest (1 or 2 points)?_____
_____

4.   What is one change I could make to reduce the stressors in my life?_____
_____

B.   **Health Enhancement:**

1.   Demonstrate two or three relaxation strategies or techniques to the class.
2.   Develop the tool and conduct a survey of people your age and profile the most common stressors in their lives. Summarize and report your findings.
3.   People cope with stress in many different ways. What fictional character deals with stressors in a similar way that you do. Give some examples.

C: **Health Promotion:**
1.   List three ways you could be involved in reducing the stress levels of the general population.
2.   List three ways cultural, environmental (physical or social-economic), political, religious, or health care attitudes/actions could be directly or indirectly involved in reducing the stress levels of the general population.
3.   Suggest one way that you personally could be a "stress reducing" advocate for each of the two target groups: (1) family; (2) friends.

Chapter Review Test

Multiple Choice: Directions: In the space at the left, write the letter of the choice that best completes each of the following statements:

_____   1. The physical or psychological response to any demand made upon the body is called: (p. 75)
   a. eustress
   b. distress
   c. adjustment
   d. stress

_____   2. The number of stages our bodies go through during Selye's General Adaptation Syndrome is: (p. 75)
   a. one
   b. two
   c. three
   d. four

_____   3. In which phase of the General Adaptation Syndrome does the body attempt to return the body to its normal state? (p.77)
   a. alarm reaction
   b. resistance
   c. fatigue
   d. exhaustion

_____   4. That phase of the General Adaptation Syndrome in which the physical and psychological energy used to fight the stressors have been depleted making one more susceptible to illness and disease is called the: (p. 77)
   a. alarm phase
   b. resistance phase
   c. fatigue phase
   d. exhaustion phase

_____   5. Good (positive) stress is referred to by Selye as: (p. 77)
   a. strain
   b. stress
   c. distress
   d. eustress

_____   6. Bad (unpleasant) stress, such as the loss of a job, is labeled by Selye as: (p. 77)
   a. strain
   b. stress
   c. distress
   d. eustress

_____   7. All of the following are examples of events that cause eustress EXCEPT: (pp. 78-79)
  a.   burn-out at work
  b.   excitement of a vacation
  c.   the accomplishment of an outstanding personal achievement
  d.   the stimulus of an exciting classroom.

_____   8. Type A personalities in contrast to Type B personalities are described as being: (p.79)
  a.   more relaxed and patient
  b.   less prone to heart disease
  c.   driven and impatient
  d.   passive and reserved

_____   9. A state of physical and mental exhaustion caused by excessive stress is called: (p. 78)
  a.   conflict
  b.   burnout
  c.   overload
  d.   pressure

_____   10. All of the following symptoms are typical of stress-related disorders with the exception of:
  (p. 81)
  a.   migraine headaches and irritability
  b.   stomach aches and skin rashes
  c.   insomnia and heart palpitations
  d.   hot flashes and sore throat

_____   11. Adaptation to stress is referred to as: (p. 85)
  a.   coping
  b.   adjusting
  c.   hardiness
  d.   quieting

_____   12. In recognizing stress exists, one must manage it effectively; a process called: (p. 86)
  a.   defense mechanization
  b.   stressor identification
  c.   personality hardiness
  d.   fight-or-flight reaction

_____   13. Interpersonal skills include all BUT which of the following examples? (p.88)
  a.   sharing feelings
  b.   active listening
  c.   passivity training
  d.   conflict resolution

_____ 14. A stress management technique that involves breathing relaxation is: (p. 90)
   a. progressive muscle relaxation
   b. meditation
   c. biofeedback
   d. stress inoculation

_____ 15. A common form of cognitive-behavioral skills training is: (p. 90)
   a. biofeedback
   b. progressive muscle relaxation
   c. meditation
   d. stress inoculation

CHAPTER 5
EATING SMART

Chapter Overview

This chapter focuses on nutrition. The chapter's objective is to promote a better understanding of what constitutes a healthy style of eating. Included is a questionnaire to test your nutritional knowledge.

What You Need to Eat: The Essential Nutrients. The body breaks down food into different chemical compounds called nutrients, which include carbohydrates, proteins, fats, vitamins, minerals, and water. Carbohydrates are divided into *simple carbohydrates*, examples being corn syrup and table sugar; and *complex carbohydrates* such as certain starches and fibers. Included is a list of foods high in fiber. Proteins are composed of chains of amino acids. *Complete proteins* contain all the amino acids. *Incomplete proteins* contain partial amounts. Fats are divided into *saturated fats*, found in animal products or certain oils, and *unsaturated fats*, which are either *polyunsaturated* or *monounsaturated*. Because margarine is high in cholesterol, the article "At Issue: Should Margarine be Shunned like Butter?" examines the pros and cons of substituting margarine for butter. The body also requires certain amounts of vitamins and minerals. A table showing the benefits of various vitamins and a diagram listing foods that contain the mineral, calcium are included.

Why Artificial Ingredients Are Added. Many different chemical compounds, called additives, are used in enhancing food products for reasons of packaging, preserving, esthetics, taste, production, and nutrient enrichment. The five types of additives are *nutrients, preservatives, processing aids, flavorings,* and *colorings*. Research suggests that many additives are potentially unhealthy.

Recommended Dietary Allowances: How Much Do You Need? The *recommended dietary allowances* (RDAs) are not hard and fast rules to follow, but should be used as guidelines after taking account of one's own physical size, lifestyle, age, and health. The new Food Guide Pyramid, shown in the chapter, is considered another good formula for daily food intake.

Eating Styles. Most eating habits are first learned from the family or ethnic group where a person was reared, yet more and more people eat out, often in fast food restaurants where the food is often not nutritious. Listed is "Your Fast-Food Sandwich Guide," which can help people make healthy choices. The **Cultural View** article explains the low fat foods to choose from in different ethnic restaurants. Vegetarians, who can be *vegans, lactovegetarians,* or *ovolactovegetarians,* omit animal products in different degrees.

How Eating Habits Become Unhealthy. . .and How to Correct That. The three most common unhealthy habits are skipping meals, excessive vitamin intake, and immoderate snacking. Understanding food terms and labels, shopping for fresh or low processed foods, and using healthy cooking methods will all contribute to healthy eating habits.

There are four **Critical Thinking Questions** interjected throughout the chapter. The first discusses whether or not high sodium intake among Americans is due to the lack of health information and asks what form of intervention public health officials should take to curb this phenomenon. The second issue examines how certain food industries can manipulate nutrition guides for their own economic benefit. The third question suggests potential problems with controlling food industries in the interest of public health. The fourth question encourages educating the young to read food labels for nutrition content.

Chapter Focus Questions

1.   What essential nutrients make up food?

2.   What are the primary sources for each nutrient and how do each contribute to overall health?

3.   What is the difference between a complete protein and an incomplete protein?

4.   How is blood cholesterol affected by diet?

5.   What types of food additives are there and how does each contribute to the quality of food?

6.   What is the purpose and function of the recommended dietary allowance (RDAs) published by the Food and Nutrition Board of the National Academy of Science?

7.   What are several eating styles and how does each contribute or detract from overall health?

8.   What common eating habits present a threat to the health of college students?

9.   How does a food label describe the nutritional value of that food?

10.   How does food preparation both enhance and detract from the quality of food?

Case Study Reflections

Fred and Antonio have widely differing dietary habits. Fred does not take the time to eat right or even consider doing so. Antonio, on the other hand, makes time to eat right and allows good sense to guide what he eats.

1.   "I know I don't eat healthy," Fred says about his diet, "but I prefer to eat what tastes good. Besides, I'll change my habits when I'm older." After reading the chapter, how would you respond to Fred's comment?

2.   Briefly identify the problem areas of Fred's diet. Because of his diet, what health problems is Fred susceptible to? With respect to the comment Fred made above, what practical dietary changes would you recommend for him?

3.   Fred and Antonio's diets radically affect the way they feel physically and mentally. How are their respective diets affecting them physically? How are their diets affecting them mentally?

4.   One of the differences between Fred and Antonio's diet is preparation. How is the food preparation in Antonio's diet better than Fred's?

Chapter Activities

A. Personal Assessment:
Am I eating smart? To find out, circle the answer that best applies to you.

		Never		Sometimes		Always
1.	I have 6-11 servings of bread, cereal, rice, or pasta daily.	1	2	3	4	5
2.	I have 2-4 servings of fruit daily.	1	2	3	4	5
3.	I have 2-3 servings of meat, poultry, fish, beans, eggs, or nuts daily.	1	2	3	4	5
4.	I have 3-5 servings of vegetables daily.	1	2	3	4	5
5.	I eat fats, oils, and sweets sparingly.	1	2	3	4	5
6.	I drink at least six to eight cups of water daily.	1	2	3	4	5
7.	I skip meals.	5	4	3	2	1
8.	I can interpret food labels.	1	2	3	4	5
9.	I know how to obtain reliable nutrition-related information, products, and services.	1	2	3	4	5

Conclusion:
1. Add up your score. The maximum score is 45. The higher the score, the more "smart eating habits" you have.

2. Which area(s) did you score the highest (4 or 5 points)? _____
_____

3. Which area(s) did you score the lowest (1 or 2 points)?_____
_____

4. What is one change I could make to improve my eating habits?_____
_____

B: Health Enhancement:

1. Go to a fast food restaurant. Observe and tabulate the food choices of customers for 30 minutes. Summarize your findings.
2. Describe several strategies that could "motivate" people toward better eating habits.

3.   How could supermarkets be designed better to assist customers in making healthier food choices?
4.   Prepare a poster describing the differing nutritional needs of special conditions such as intense athletics, pregnancy, elderly, children and adolescents.
5.   Gather menus from several culturally diverse restaurants. Make nutritional comparisons.

C: Health Promotion:

1.   List three ways you could be involved in improving the smart eating habits of the general population.
2.   List three ways cultural, environmental (physical or social-economic), political, religious, or health care attitudes/actions could be directly or indirectly involved in improving the smart eating habits of the general population.
3.   Suggest one way that you personally could be a "smart eating habits" advocate for each of the two target groups: (1) family; (2) friends.

Chapter Review Test

Multiple Choice: Directions: In the space at the left write the letter of the choice that best completes each of the following statements.

_____   1. The nutrients that provide our bodies with calories include all of the following EXCEPT: (p. 97)
a. carbohydrates
b. proteins
c. fats
d. minerals

_____   2. The basic chemical compounds in food that are required for growth are referred to as: (p. 97)
a. nutrients
b. amino acids
c. dietology
d. cellulose

_____   3. The body's primary source of energy comes from: (p. 97)
a. carbohydrates
b. vitamins
c. proteins
d. minerals

_____   4. Carbohydrates primarily found in whole grains, fruits and vegetables are called: (p. 97)
a. simple carbohydrates
b. complex carbohydrates
c. sucrose
d. glucose

_____   5. Common examples of complex carbohydrates are: (p. 98)
a. starches and fiber
b. sucrose and dextrose
c. vitamins and minerals
d. phosphates and nitrates

_____   6. Dietary fiber is commonly defined as: (p. 98)
a. any food that is digested by enzymes in the small intestines
b. any food that is digested and absorbed into the bloodstream
c. the roughage that is digested in the small intestine
d. the part of the food that is not digested but rather aids in the movement of bowels

_____ 7. Food that contains all nine of the essential amino acids such as those found in animal products is referred to as: (p. 100)
    a. essential amino acids
    b. nonessential amino acids
    c. complete proteins
    d. incomplete proteins

_____ 8. Fats found in animal products and suspected of promoting cardiovascular disease are called: (p. 100)
    a. saturated
    b. unsaturated
    c. polyunsaturated
    d. monounsaturated

_____ 9. These fats are found in high quantities in peanut and olive oils: (p. 100)
    a. saturated
    b. unsaturated
    c. polyunsaturated
    d. monounsaturated

_____ 10. This fat-like substance, manufactured by the liver, is necessary for the formation of bodily process such as the formation of sex hormones, vitamin D and bile. (p. 100)
    a. glycerol
    b. cholesterol
    c. fatty acid
    d. triglyceride

_____ 11. Compounds that transport cholesterol in the bloodstream to the liver where it is used to produce bile are called: (p. 100)
    a. plaque
    b. monounsaturated fats
    c. high density lipoproteins
    d. low density lipoproteins

_____ 12. The build-up of cholesterol in the walls of the arteries is also called: (p. 101)
    a. plaque
    b. glycerols
    c. triglyceride
    d. fiber

_____ 13. Water-soluble vitamins must be consumed daily because: (p. 102)
    a. they are not stored by the body
    b. amounts not used by the body are excreted in urine
    c. they are stored by the body's fat cell
    d. a and b only

_____   14. A disorder in which bone density decreases and bones are more likely to break is called: (p. 104)
    a. arthritis
    b. atherosclerosis
    c. osteoporosis
    d. osteoarthritis

_____   15. Additives are added to our food for all of the following reasons EXCEPT to: (p. 107)
    a. change the food flavor
    b. enhance the quality of food
    c. make food more attractive
    d. maintain food freshness

CHAPTER 6
MAINTAINING PROPER WEIGHT

Chapter Overview

This chapter describes why a healthy weight is necessary for overall good health, how to determine and manage one's proper weight, and the problems, diseases and concerns associated with weight control.

How Weight Can Be Harmful to Your Health. *Obesity* involves an excess of body fat, but, to be *overweight* is to have an overall higher weight than what is average for your height. Both extremes cause health problems, especially hypertension. To be *underweight* is also determined according to one's height and can cause health problems, or be a symptom, as in *anorexia*.

Assessing Weight. Some of the ways to evaluate one's weight is using height-weight charts, body mass index, or measuring body fat which can be done using methods such as: *the pinch test, underwater weighing*, or *bioelectrical impedance*. What is perceived as a correct weight is often determined by society. The **Cultural View** article, "How You See Yourself Can Depend on the Culture of the Time," gives examples of how most normal weight people are concerned with losing or gaining weight in order to obtain a cultural ideal.

Why Do Some People Get Fat? Although some people gain weight from endocrine-related diseases, most obesity is related to genetics, learned eating behaviors, poor exercise habits, or emotional problems.

How the Body Stores and Uses Energy. Food provides the body with energy; some of the leftover food that is not burned for energy is stored as fat, which can be utilized later. A *calorie* is a unit used to measure the amount of energy burned. Although, high caloric intake is related to weight gain, more calories should come from carbohydrates than fat. Moderate amounts of fat are necessary to absorb essential vitamins, but the less calories that come from fat, the less the chance for high weight gain. To reach and then maintain a healthy weight, exercise is a necessary component to healthy eating.

Eating Disorders: A Troubled Relationship with Food. *Anorexia* is a disease when the afflicted person attempts to loose weight through starvation. A *binge eating disorder* is when a person eats excessive amounts of food in one setting until they are extremely uncomfortable; whereas, *bulimia* involves binge eating, but is immediately followed by a purging of the food. People who suffer from these disorders often have low-self esteem, lack of control and a fear of being fat. Included in the chapter is a questionnaire to determine if you are at risk for an eating disorder.

Reality of Weight Control. Instead of trying to lose weight with a diet, you should try to improve your diet with healthier, more balanced meals supplementing this with exercise. Fad diets, especially those that insist on a lack of carbohydrates or protein and/or include fasting, should be avoided because ultimately they fail to produce weight loss and can instead cause other health problems as suggested in the accompanying article, "Questions to Ask Before Going on a Diet."

Developing Healthskills article, "How Not to Gain Weight When You Eat Low-Fat Foods," explains that many people overeat if given low-fat food.

Interjected throughout the chapter are four **Critical Thinking Questions** which explore: (1) the usefulness of monitoring weight with a bathroom scale; (2) the societal and economic causes that may occur with a significant reduction in overweight people; (3) the connection between nutrition education and weight control; and (4) the proliferation of the fad diet industry despite the lack of health benefits for the consumer.

Chapter Focus Questions

1. What are the benefits of maintaining normal weight and the health risks associated with overweight?

2. What are the health risks of being underweight?

3. How might one assess his/her body weight, as well as approximate body mass?

4. Why do some people become overweight more easily than others?

5. How do eating behaviors influence body composition, and how are eating behaviors learned?

6. For what reasons is fat in the diet essential for health, and why does excess fat lead to health risks?

7. What is the relationship between exercise and weight control?

8. What is the nature of anorexia and bulimia?

9. What ways are there to control your weight and maintain health?

10. How can fad diets be harmful to your health?

Case Study Reflections

Sara and Kisha have had weight problems for a considerable period of time. Although each has tried many quick weight-loss diets, only Kisha has found long-term success, while Sarah continues to feel only frustration in her attempts to lose weight.

1.   After reading the chapter, what factors motivate Sarah to lose weight? How much weight does she want to lose? Is her goal realistic or even healthy?

2   Both Sarah and Kisha have tried several different diets. Why might these diets work in the short term but often fail in the long term? What nutritional drawbacks are there to these diets?

3.   As a friend of yours, Sarah mentions to you how discouraged she is about her weight-loss. What encouragement would you give her? What factors regarding weight loss are beyond her control?

4.   Kisha's last diet has become her "life-long diet." What does this mean in terms of eating habits? How important is exercise to this "life-long diet?"

Chapter Activities

A: **Personal Assessment:**
Am I maintaining my proper weight? To find out, circle the answer that best applies to you.

		Never		Sometimes		Always
1.	My body mass index is in the healthy zone.	1	2	3	4	5
2.	My body fat ratio is within a healthy range.	1	2	3	4	5
3.	When I look in the mirror, I look overweight.	5	4	3	2	1
4.	I feel overweight.	5	4	3	2	1
5.	Obesity and overweight is in my genetic background.	5	4	3	2	1
6.	My family traditions support healthy eating.	1	2	3	4	5
7.	My cultural influences support healthy eating.	1	2	3	4	5
8.	I am "in tune" with my hunger.	1	2	3	4	5
9.	I am preoccupied with "thinness."	5	4	3	2	1
10.	I often go on crash diets.	5	4	3	2	1
11.	I know how to obtain reliable weight-related information, products, and services.	1	2	3	4	5

Conclusion:
1.   Add up your score. The maximum score is 55. The higher the score, the more "proper weight" literate you are.

2.   Which area(s) did you score the highest (4 or 5 points)?_____
_____

3.   Which area(s) did you score the lowest (1 or 2 points)?_____
_____

4.   What is one change I could make to maintain/improve my proper weight?_____
_____

B.   Health Enhancement:

1.   Research to find a formula used to estimate the number of daily calories an individual needs to maintain his/her present weight. Use this formula for yourself and compare to the actual number of daily calories.
2.   Design a three-day menu for an individual with special dietary restrictions.
3.   Compare two or more popular national weight-loss diets/programs.

C.   Health Promotion:

1.   List three ways you could be involved in helping the general population achieve and maintain proper weight.
2.   List three ways cultural, environmental (physical or social-economic), political, religious, or health care attitudes/actions could be directly or indirectly involved in improving the achievement and maintenance of proper weight in the general population.
3.   Suggest one way that you personally could be a "proper weight advocate" for each of the two target groups: (1) family; (2) friends.

Chapter Review Test

Multiple Choice: Directions: In the space at the left write the letter of the choice that best completes each of the following statements:

_____   1. Obesity is a synonym for: (p.127)
- a. overweight
- b. non-essential fat
- c. weighty
- d. essential fat

_____   2. Obese people are more likely than their non-obese peers to suffer from all BUT which of the following health problems? (p.127)
- a. elevated blood cholesterol levels
- b. cardiovascular diseases
- c. adult-onset diabetes
- d. arthritis

_____   3. The Framingham Study reports that the chance of sudden death from heart attack is more than three times as great for people who are _____ percent overweight. (p. 128)
- a. 5
- b. 10
- c. 15
- d. 20

_____   4. Low body fat in females is implicated in: (p.128)
- a. amenorrhea
- b. dysmenorrhea
- c. apnea
- d. hyperthyroidism

_____   5. Experts caution against relying too much on height and weight tables alone for all BUT which of the following reasons? (p. 129)
- a. They are not applicable to the entire population.
- b. They ignore other risk factors such as age and activity levels.
- c. They do not measure the distribution of fat in the body.
- d. They do not consider body shape and size.

_____   6. A body mass index assesses the: (p. 131)
- a. essential fat to storage fat ratio
- b. relationship of strength to power
- c. relationship of body weight to height
- d. fat to muscle ratio

_____   7. The pinch test measuring technique (p. 131)
   a. is used to measure muscle mass
   b. measures subcutaneous fat in various places on the body
   c. is a more accurate way to measure percent of body fat than other techniques
   d. is used to measure essential fat stores

_____   8. Determining body fat utilizing small electrodes attached to a person's wrists and ankles to measure the body's water content is called: (p. 131)
   a. body mass index
   b. pinch test
   c. bioelectrical impedance
   d. hydrostatic immersion

_____   9. Determining body fat by measuring the amount of water displaced when a person is completely submerged is called: (p. 131)
   a. body mass index
   b. pinch test
   c. bioelectrical impedance
   d. hydrostatic immersion

_____   10. The set point theory suggests that the body knows when it: (p. 135)
   a. cannot lose more weight
   b. is nearest its best height
   c. is nearest its best weight
   d. requires more food intake

_____   11. Childhood obesity is influenced by all BUT which of the following factors? (p. 135)
   a. parent's weight, age, and marital status
   b. socioeconomic class
   c. race/ethnicity
   d. region of country lived in

_____   12. The normal range of body fat for the healthy young woman is: (p. 139)
   a. 10-15%
   b. 17-20%
   c. 23-26%
   d. 27-30%

_____   13. The speed with which the body expends calories on basic functions such as respiration and circulation is referred to as: (p. 139)
   a. basal metabolic rate
   b. resting metabolic rate
   c. exercise metabolic rate
   d. body mass rate

_____   14. Taken together, calorie requirements decrease ____ to ____ percent for each decade of life past age 20. (p. 140)
   a.   2-8
   b.   12-18
   c.   20-26
   d.   32-38

_____   15. An eating disorder characterized by the extreme behavior of binge eating and purging is called: (p. 141)
   a.   anorexia nervosa
   b.   bulimia
   c.   binge eating disorder
   d.   compulsive eating disorder

CHAPTER 7
KEEPING FIT

Chapter Overview

This chapter concentrates on promoting physical activity for all people, not just athletes. Discussion centers on how to correctly determine the proper level of physical fitness, explain various exercises and their benefits, as well as instruct on how to incorporate an exercise program into daily life so physical wellness can be habitually and actively maintained.

Who is Exercising? Participation in exercise varies according to demographic groups, but physical activity habits learned as a child often carry through into adulthood. Gender is also a determining factor as an accompanying table shows what percentage of young adults engage in what types of exercise.

Health Benefits of Exercise. Many researchers believe exercise is the most important aspect of a healthy life. Exercise reduces risks of heart disease and strengthens the heart's functionality, prevents osteoporosis, improves the immune system, reduces weight, and can positively affect mental health. A table shows the average amount of calories burned during certain exercise activities.

Fitness Triangle. *Physical fitness* measures how well your body is working. To keep the body functioning to its potential three essential elements must be met through exercise: *strength, flexibility* and *endurance*. A checklist shows how you can determine your flexibility.

Fitness Through Exercise. To exercise productively, you need to work out intensively enough to raise the heart rate to a safe, yet, higher level, engage in an exercise that lasts for a proper duration and exercise frequently. The article, "Starting Out: A Walking Program," suggests, especially for beginners, walking for a simple and safe exercise regimen.

Skills for Planning and Maintaining a Personal Fitness Program. Before beginning an exercise program, you need to assess your fitness level which can be done by monitoring your heart rate and by visiting a physician. Any physical activity should begin with a *warm-up*, followed by the *conditioning period*, then finish with a *cool-down*. To reduce the risk of injury during exercise, it is necessary to be cautious and well-informed. The short essay, "A Timeline for Self-Treatment of Exercise Injuries," explains how to treat minor injuries using the RICE method (rest, ice, compression, and elevation). Good exercise equipment can be indispensable as the example shown in the **Healthwise Consumer** article, "The Right Shoe For You." illustrates. Most importantly start an exercise program, even if in the beginning the activity is minimal. Listed are many moderate activities that can count as exercise.

Interspersed throughout the chapter are four **Critical Thinking Questions** which examine: (1) the importance of physical education in schools; (2) the difficulties in measuring mental health benefits gained from exercise; (3) the potential benefits of a workplace fitness program for both employee and employer; and (4) how to remove the obstacles that keep people from a disciplined exercise program.

Chapter Focus Questions

1.   To what extent do people exercise and for what reasons are there low levels of exercise among specific populations?

2.   What are the physical health benefits of exercise?

3.   What is the effect of exercise on psychological well-being?

4.   How would you explain the following three major components of fitness: strength, flexibility and endurance?

5.   What is the difference between isokinetic, isotonic and isometric exercises?

6.   What is the difference between aerobic and anaerobic activities?

7.   What is the importance of intensity, duration and frequency of exercise sessions?

8.   What procedures are followed when determining your target heart rate for exercise as well as your maximal heart rate?

9.   What considerations should be kept in mind when planning a personal fitness program including warm-up, conditioning and cool-down periods?

10. How would you describe the tactics necessary for maintaining a fitness program?

Case Study Reflections

Chapter seven opens by comparing the exercise plans of Gilda and Toshio. Gilda exercises vigorously on the weekends with various activities. Toshio takes a more balanced approach to exercise, following a weekly schedule and building regular exercise into the day.

1. After reading the chapter, list the physical benefits and/or drawbacks that both Gilda and Toshio experience in their exercise program. Whose exercise plan is better? Why?

2. Is there a psychological difference between the two exercise programs? Explain.

3. "Gilda's exercise program is better because she's doing what she loves when she wants to do it." Is this an accurate statement? Why or why not?

4. Considering Gilda's current exercise patterns, create a more balanced exercise program that you think would work for her. What will it take for her to "stick with it"?

Chapter Activities

A.   Personal Assessment:

Am I keeping fit? To find out, circle the answer that best applies to you.

		Never		Sometimes		Always
1	Exercise has a high priority in my life.	1	2	3	4	5
2.	I participate in muscular strength building exercises.	1	2	3	4	5
3.	I participate in stretching exercises.	1	2	3	4	5
4.	I participate in muscular endurance exercises.	1	2	3	4	5
5.	I participate in cardiovascular strengthening exercises.	1	2	3	4	5
6.	I can distinguish between aerobic and anaerobic exercises.	1	2	3	4	5
7.	I can name several benefits of exercise.	1	2	3	4	5
8.	I measure my heart rate in order to indicate exercise intensity.	1	2	3	4	5
9.	I exercise in my target heart rate at least three times per week for 30 minutes.	1	2	3	4	5
10.	I do warm-up activities before I exercise.	1	2	3	4	5
11.	I do cool-down activities after I exercise.	1	2	3	4	5
12.	I avoid injuries when I exercise.	1	2	3	4	5
13.	I exercise in a safe environment.	1	2	3	4	5
14.	I know how to obtain reliable exercise-related information, products, and services.	1	2	3	4	5

Conclusion:

1.   Add up your score. The maximum score is 70. The higher the score, the more "exercise" literate you are.

2.   Which area(s) did you score the highest (4 or 5 points)?_____
_____

3.   Which area(s) did you score the lowest (1 or 2 points)?_____
_____

4.   What is one change I could make to improve my exercise habits? _____
_____

B.   Health Enhancement:

1.   Compare several popular professional sports in terms of the level of fitness necessary for participation.
2.   Design a fitness program for an individual with a physical disability.
3.   Identify and rank several common physical activities in terms of physical benefit.
4.   Make a chart or poster illustrating cultural similarities and differences related to physical activities.

C.   Health Promotion:

1.   List three ways you could be involved in helping the general population achieve and maintain improved fitness levels.
2.   List three ways cultural, environmental (physical or social-economic), political, religious, or health care attitudes/actions could be directly or indirectly involved in improving the fitness levels in the general population.
3.   Suggest one way that you personally could be a "fitness" advocate for each of the two target groups: (1) family; (2) friends.

Chapter Review Test

Multiple choice: Directions: In the space at the left, write the letter of the choice that best completes each of the following statements.

_____ 1. Which of the following is NOT one of the health-related benefits of regular exercise? (pp. 155-156)
   a. reduces the risk of coronary artery disease
   b. reduces the risk of hypertension
   c. helps control weight
   d. reduces the risk of colon cancer

_____ 2. Strengthening bones as a benefit of exercise reduces the risk for: (p. 158)
   a. osteo-arthritis
   b. osteoporosis
   c. rheumatoid arthritis
   d. Osgood-Schlaters

_____ 3. The so-called runners high or a feeling of euphoria when exercising is due to the effect of this hormone. (p. 160)
   a. adrenalin
   b. nor-adrenalin
   c. endorphin
   d. serotonin

_____ 4. Mental health benefits of exercise include all the of the following EXCEPT: (pp. 160-161)
   a. less anxiety
   b. greater job satisfaction
   c. better self-esteem
   d. dramatic mood swings

_____ 5. Strength development exercises in which a weight is moved through a full range of motion are called: (p. 163)
   a. isokinetic
   b. isotonic
   c. isometric
   d. isobionic

_____ 6. The ability to move joints through their normal range of motion is a measure of: (p. 163)
   a. strength
   b. flexibility
   c. muscular endurance
   d. agility

_____ 7. The volume of oxygen that the body can consume in one minute of exercise is referred to as: (p. 163)
   a. strength
   b. flexibility
   c. muscular endurance
   d. aerobic capacity

_____ 8. Strength development exercises that require muscles to contract against immovable objects are called: (p. 163)
   a. isokinetic
   b. isotonic
   c. isometric
   d. isobionic

_____ 9. Anaerobic literally means: (p. 165)
   a. less anxious
   b. isotonic
   c. with oxygen
   d. without oxygen

_____ 10. The best overall indicator of exercise intensity is: (p. 165)
   a. respiratory rate
   b. heart rate
   c. body weight
   d. aerobic capacity

_____ 11. According to the Surgeon General, the number of times per week a person should exercise is: (p. 165)
   a. one-two
   b. two-three
   c. three-four
   d. three-five

_____ 12. The number of times per week exercise is needed to achieve a training effect is known as: (p. 165)
   a. frequency
   b. duration
   c. intensity
   d. repetition

_____ 13. The improvement in one's heart from regular exercise is known as the : (p. 166)
   a. training effect
   b. intensity effect
   c. aerobic effect
   d. target heart rate

_____   14. Heart activity high enough to bring about a training effect and low enough to be safe is referred to as: (p. 167)
    a.   maximal heart rate
    b.   sub-maximal heart rate
    c.   aerobic capacity rate
    d.   target heart rate

_____   15. Tactics necessary for maintaining a regular active fitness program include which of the following? (pp. 167-168)
    a.   set a regular time and place to exercise
    b.   establish realistic goals that can be achieved
    c.   alternate the physical activities within the program
    d.   all of the above

CHAPTER 8
SMOKING OUT TOBACCO

Chapter Overview

Although, there is much public awareness of the dangerous chemicals in cigarettes, many people still smoke. This chapter examines the power of the tobacco addiction, and explains the numerous health problems related to tobacco use, concentrating on cigarette smoking and the benefits gained from quitting.

Who Smokes? Studies show that certain demographic trends, such as race, gender, education, income level, and age are factors when trying to compile the profile of a smoker. These trends have changed throughout history; listed is a chart showing today's current smokers. People who smoke tend to have other poor health habits as well.

Why People Smoke. People begin to smoke and continue the habit due to parental and peer influences, convincing advertising campaigns, feelings of pleasure and relaxation from smoking, and the nicotine addiction. There are several similar characteristics between tobacco addiction and other drug addictions, such as heroin and cocaine.

The Components of Cigarette Smoke. When inhaling, 90% of the *nicotine* in cigarettes is absorbed into the bloodstream which induces the release of epinephrine and adrenaline, while increasing the heart's workload. *Tar* is one of the many dangerous *carcinogens* (a toxic chemical) found in a cigarette. Cigarettes also contain high levels of the gas, *carbon monoxide*, which interferes with the movement of oxygen throughout the body. A questionnaire is inserted to test your knowledge of the physical effects of smoking.

Why Smoking is Dangerous to Your Health. Smoking is the leading cause of lung cancer and is an attributable factor in developing other cancers, heart disease, strokes, emphysema, chronic bronchitis, other lung diseases and infections, complications for pregnant mothers and developing fetuses, SIDS, allergies, cataracts, digestive and circulatory diseases, protracted healing of wounds, and wrinkles! Tables and graphs in this section show the health care expenditures for smoking-related illnesses, the risks of lung cancer for smokers and non-smokers, as well as the positive effects of smoking cessation on lung cancer. The **Healthwise Consumer** article addresses the pros and cons of smoking low-tar, low-nicotine cigarettes.

How Noncigarette Smokers Are Exposed to Tobacco. *Sidestream* smoke, the smoke from the end of a cigarette that is not inhaled by the smoker, is a health hazard for nonsmokers. Cigars, pipe and smokeless tobacco contain carcinogens that cause mouth cancer as well as other oral diseases. A guideline to self detect disease for smokeless tobacco users is included in the chapter.

Kicking the Habit: How to Stop. As only about 10% of smokers are successful in quitting, smoking is one of the most difficult addictions to conquer, yet many people find a motivation to try to quit. Both the physical and psychological symptoms of withdrawal can be quite disturbing, but *smoking cessation* assistance is available in forms of *behavior modification*, *nicotine replacement*, and hypnosis. Included is a list of activities assisting ex-smokers to avoid tobacco. The **Cultural View** article tells how a whole village in Fiji was successful in quitting smoking because they religiously forbade the use of tobacco.

The Changing Climate on Public Acceptance of Tobacco Use. The increase in the awareness of the harmful effects of cigarette smoking over the last several years has been evidenced via legislation, social pressures and public health policy. By reading the historical events related to tobacco in the **Tobacco Timeline,** you can mark the change in the American public's attitude regarding smoking.

There are four **Critical Thinking Questions** throughout the chapter. These questions focus on: (1) what may be the most effective methods in preventing young people from beginning to smoke; (2) who should be held financially responsible for smoking related illnesses; (3) the ethics of cigarette taxation; and (4) whether the tobacco industries should pay for smoking related health care for recipients of Medicaid.

Chapter Focus Questions

1. How would you describe the typical smoker and what are his/her reasons for choosing to use tobacco?

2. What are the similarities of dependence on tobacco products and drug addiction?

3. How has advertising influenced the rate of tobacco use?

4. What is passive smoke and what is the risk associated with this involuntary exposure to tobacco?

5. What are three major components of cigarette smoke and their health risk?

6. How does tobacco use contribute to cancer, heart disease and lung disease?

7. What effect does smoking have on the developing fetus of a pregnant woman?

8. What assertive techniques can be used to avoid tobacco use?

9. How might you differentiate and compare the effects of smoking and the use of smokeless tobacco?

10. What are the three means of smoking cessation described in your textbook and what are their comparative advantages?

Case Study Reflections

In the opening to chapter 8, Manuel is unable to resist his "need" for a cigarette while driving and late for school. Donetta, meanwhile, does resist her desire for a cigarette even though she is out with friends who smoke.

1.   Do Manuel and Donetta's respective situations or environments influence their decision to smoke or not smoke? How? Why?

2.   What physiological and psychological "needs" make Manuel and Donetta want to smoke?

3.   Should Manuel take a different approach the next time he tries to quit? If so, what approach should be taken?

4.   What do you think was the most important factor in Donetta's ability to quit? Why?

Chapter Activities

A.   Personal Assessment:
Am I "smoking out tobacco?" To find out, circle the answer that best applies to you.

		Never		Sometimes		Always
1.	I smoke for pleasure.	5	4	3	2	1
2.	I smoke for relaxation.	5	4	3	2	1
3.	I am addicted to smoking.	5	4	3	2	1
4.	Smoking makes me feel better.	5	4	3	2	1
5.	I have tried unsuccessfully to quit smoking.	5	4	3	2	1
6.	When I don't smoke I suffer from withdrawal symptoms.	5	4	3	2	1
7.	I can refuse a cigarette when offered.	1	2	3	4	5
8.	I have experienced a smoking-related illness.	5	4	3	2	1
9.	I am exposed to sidestream smoke.	5	4	3	2	1
10.	I am exposed to mainstream smoke.	5	4	3	2	1
11.	I use smokeless (chewing or snuff) tobacco.	5	4	3	2	1
12.	I know how to obtain reliable smoking-related information, products, and service.	1	2	3	4	5

Conclusion:

1.   Add up your score. The maximum score is 60. The higher the score, the more "smoking out tobacco" literate you are.

2.   Which area(s) did you score the highest (4 or 5 points)?_____
_____

3.   Which area(s) did you score the lowest (1 or 2 points)?_____
_____

4.   What is one change I could make to improve my "smoking out tobacco" literacy?_____
_____

B.   Health Enhancement:

1.   Calculate the cost of tobacco use over several years. Using periodic benchmarks (e.g.: 5 years, 8 years, etc.), make a chart or poster illustrating "healthier" choices that a similar amount of money could purchase.

2.   Survey several restaurants to determine the percentage of "space" designated as non-smoking space. Summarize your findings and share with the class.

3.   Research to find out connections, generally unknown to the public, that several of the tobacco companies have to common non-tobacco products, services, or organizations.

4.   Develop a chart or poster that illustrates the immediate and long-term effect of tobacco use.

5.   Compare several national quit smoking programs and products.

C.   Health Promotion:

1.   List three ways you could be involved in helping to reduce the incidence of smoking in the general population.

2.   List three ways cultural, environmental (physical or social-economic), political, religious, or health care attitudes/actions could be directly or indirectly involved in reducing the incidence of smoking in the general population.

3.   Suggest one way that you personally could be a "no smoking" advocate for each of the two target groups: (1) family; (2) friends.

Chapter Review Test

Multiple Choice: In the space at the left, write the letter of the choice that best completes each of the following statements.

_____   1. Which of the following situation(s) makes a person smoke that first cigarette and continue to smoke? (p. 181)
   a.   influences from family and friends
   b.   the allure of advertisements
   c.   the addictive nature of tobacco
   d.   all of the above

_____   2. Which of the following parental influences is least likely to result in a teenager's decision not to smoke? (p. 181)
   a.   restrictiveness and harsh criticism
   b.   affection
   c.   emotional support
   d.   meaningful conversations

_____   3. Research indicates that smoking a cigarette causes the blood pressure and heart rate to: (p. 183)
   a.   increase
   b.   decrease
   c.   remain the same
   d.   rise and decrease respectively

_____   4. The psychoactive agent found naturally in tobacco and responsible for the addictive behavior of tobacco smokers is: (p. 183)
   a.   tar
   b.   nicotine
   c.   hydrocarbon
   d.   carbon monoxide

_____   5. Failure of a drug to cause the usual effect or when a higher dose is required to bring about the desired effect is referred to as: (p. 183)
   a.   tolerance
   b.   physical dependence
   c.   psychological dependence
   d.   addiction

_____   6. The carcinogens in tobacco smoke are located in the: (p. 185)
   a.   nicotine
   b.   tar
   c.   carbon monoxide
   d.   carbon dioxide

_____ 7. Carbon monoxide reduces the red blood cell's ability to transport oxygen by: (p. 185)
   a. destroying oxygen molecules
   b. thinning the blood
   c. attaching itself to hemoglobin
   d. displacing fluid in cells

_____ 8. Cigarette smoking is responsible for approximately one out of every ____ deaths in the United States. (p. 185)
   a. 5
   b. 10
   c. 15
   d. 20

_____ 9. The leading cause of cancer death from smoking among both men and women is: (p.186)
   a. stomach cancer
   b. throat cancer
   c. colon cancer
   d. lung cancer

_____ 10. All BUT which of the following are examples of carcinogenic compounds found in cigarette smoke? (p. 186)
   a. ethylene oxide
   b. ethanol
   c. styrene
   d. benzopyrene

_____ 11. Two major components in smoke that contribute to heart disease are: (p. 190)
   a. carbon monoxide and carbon dioxide
   b. carbon monoxide and nicotine
   c. nicotine and tar
   d. ash and hydrocarbons

_____ 12. Women who smoke and use birth control pills are at increased risk of: (p. 190)
   a. carbon monoxide poisoning
   b. chronic obstructive lung disease
   c. cervical cancer
   d. strokes and heart attacks

_____ 13. What two respiratory diseases are associated with smoking? (p. 190)
   a. chronic bronchitis and emphysema
   b. pneumonia and strokes
   c. lung cancer and pneumonia
   d. lobar pneumonia and double pneumonia

_____ 14. Which of the following statements is TRUE regarding smoking during pregnancy? (pp. 190-191)
   a. Babies born to mothers who smoke weigh less at birth than do other babies.
   b. Babies born to mothers who smoke have a higher risk of becoming obese as adults.
   c. Babies born to mothers who smoke have a higher IQ (intelligence quotient).
   d. Babies born to mothers who smoke are more likely to have genetic predispositions for high cholesterol.

_____ 15. A condition characterized by white patches on the inside of the mouth that are caused by the carcinogens in smokeless tobacco is called: (p. 193)
   a. gingivitis
   b. leukoplakia
   c. oral cancer
   d. periodontal disease

CHAPTER 9
DEALING WITH DRINKING

Chapter Overview

This chapter explains the myriad of problems that occur with the abuse of alcohol including health risks, social implications and the disease of alcoholism. It concentrates on how the individual can learn skills in order to prevent and control problem drinking.

Who Drinks: A Picture of Alcohol Consumption. About 60% of adults drink alcohol, with differences occurring between men and women, working and stay-at-home women, and the elderly. College adults drink more than any other adult group and are among the highest number of *binge drinkers*. Adolescents who are heavy drinkers have a high potential to become alcoholics.

Why Do People Drink? People consume alcohol for social reasons such as peer pressure and the belief that drinking will enhance interpersonal relationships. Listed in the text are many reasons college students give for drinking alcohol. Alcohol use is also a historical tradition for many different ethnic and religious groups. When a person's *alcohol dependence* becomes severe, they may develop an *alcohol addiction*.

Health Hazards of Alcohol. Moderate alcohol consumption is often regarded as a healthy habit, yet, the **Cultural View** article explains how the belief that the French gain health benefits from drinking red wine is problematic. Alcohol is high in calories, but the amount depends on the type of drink. Included is a list that gives an approximate calorie measure for different alcoholic beverages. Drinking affects the central nervous system by altering the functions of the *cerebrum, cerebral cortex, cerebellum and medulla*. This results in a slowing down of different body processes. The misuse of alcohol can produce *cirrhosis of the liver*, cause *fetal alcohol syndrome* in fetuses, and alcohol poisoning which ceases respiratory functions, often leading to death. Death from alcohol is most likely to occur as a result of alcohol-related traffic accidents. Attached is an article describing both the citizen groups, MADD and SADD, who have tried to eliminate drunk driving and a graph showing the decline in alcohol-related motor vehicle deaths from 1987-1994.

Alcoholism As a Disease. The definition of alcoholism includes both factors of environment and genetics, as well as psychosocial influences. Alcohol is considered a chronic disease, with compounding symptoms that can lead to death. Treatment is available to both *alcoholics*, who have no control over their drinking; and to *problem drinkers*, who exert some control over alcohol consumption but often abuse it. Included is a Self-Assessment questionnaire to determine if you misuse alcohol.

Controlling Access to Alcohol through legislation, age-limits, taxation and other public policy methods, has not proven very successful in reducing the abuses of alcohol-related behavior.

Skills to Avoid Problem Drinking. People control their drinking by either *total abstinence,* or through *situational abstinence*. When you do drink, you should pace your drinking; e.g. try not to drink on an empty stomach, avoid other drugs, and be socially assertive and aware of risky situations. To help monitor drinking, a table is included showing how to measure intoxication by the number of drinks consumed.

Prevention: The Ultimate Answer. To reduce the rate of alcoholism among adults, early prevention with young people may be one of the most important methods of prevention, taking into account family genetics and environmental factors.

There are four **Critical Thinking Questions** interjected throughout the chapter. They discuss: (1) how to curb heavy drinking habits of college students; (2) the ethical concerns of using legislative methods to control drinking in pregnant women; (3) enforcing stiffer blood alcohol limits to reduce traffic accidents; and (4) the efficacy of severe legislation, like Prohibition, to control substances.

Chapter Focus Questions

1.   How would you differentiate between the drinking patterns of the adult population, college students and adolescents?

2.   For what reasons do people drink alcohol?

3.   What is the difference between the occasional drinker, the social drinker and the problem drinker?

4.   What are the dangers of binge drinking?

5.   What are the health hazards of alcohol use and abuse?

6.   What is the relationship of alcohol use to the incidence of suicide, homicide and unintentional injuries?

7.   How is alcoholism defined as a disease?

8.   What are some treatment options for alcoholism?

9.   How might one avoid problem drinking when using social assertiveness skills?

10. Why is prevention the ultimate answer to the problems associated with alcohol use?

Case Study Reflections

In the beginning of the chapter, Fiona and William host a "bring-your-own" party that only leads to chaos and stress. On the other hand, Lois and Eduardo host a costume party where no one gets drunk and everyone leaves after having had a good time.

1.   Short of eliminating the use of alcohol at Fiona and William's party, is there a way they could have prevented the party from getting out of control? If so, what? If not, why not?

2.   After a few days, William plans to go to another party. Fiona reminds him of the disaster at last weekend's party. William says as long as he doesn't drink every night he'll be fine. After reading the chapter, what is wrong with William's logic? If you were Fiona, what would your response be?

3.   Consider Lois and Eduardo's party. Is it a realistic situation for most college students when at a party? Why, if Lois and Eduardo's party is considered successful, is alcohol so common at many college parties?

4.   Over time it becomes apparent to William that he has a problem with alcohol. His grades are failing and all he wants to do is drink. Describe William's drinking problem. What would you suggest William do to curb or stop his drinking?

Chapter Activities

Personal Assessment:

Am I "dealing with drinking?" To find out, circle the answer that best applies to you.

		Never		Sometimes		Always
1.	I am addicted to alcohol.	5	4	3	2	1
2.	Drinking alcohol makes me feel better.	5	4	3	2	1
3.	When I don't drink alcohol I suffer from withdrawal symptoms.	5	4	3	2	1
4.	I can easily refuse an alcoholic drink when offered.	1	2	3	4	5
5.	I have experienced a drinking-related illness.	5	4	3	2	1
6.	I have experienced an alcohol-related legal consequence.	5	4	3	2	1
7.	I have experienced an alcohol-related social problem.	5	4	3	2	1
8.	I have experienced an alcohol-related blackout.	5	4	3	2	1
9.	I have alcohol-related hangovers.	5	4	3	2	1
10.	I drive when my blood alcohol concentration is over .05.	5	4	3	2	1
11.	I know how to obtain reliable alcohol-related information, products, and services.	1	2	3	4	5

Conclusion:

1.   Add up your score. The maximum score is 55. The higher the score, the more "alcohol healthy" you are.

2.   Which area(s) did you score the highest (4 or 5 points)?_____
_____

3.   Which area(s) did you score the lowest (1 or 2 points)?_____
_____

4.   What is one change I could make to improve my "alcohol health" literacy?_____
_____

B.   Health Enhancement:

1.   Myth or Reality? Daily consumption of alcohol will reduce the risk of cardiovascular disease. Research and report findings to class.
2.   Myth or Reality? Alcoholism is hereditary. Research and report findings to class.
3.   Research to find out the extent that alcohol is involved in car crashes, domestic violence, and unplanned pregnancies.
4.   Write a 30 second radio commercial designed to reduce problems related to alcohol use.
5.   Provide a written response: Since alcoholism is considered, by many, a disease, can an individual use "alcoholism" as a legal defense in the same manner that another would use "mental illness?" Why or why not?

C.   Health Promotion:

1.   List three ways you could be involved in helping to reduce the incidence of harmful alcohol use in the general population.
2.   List three ways cultural, environmental (physical or social-economic), political, religious, or health care attitudes/actions could be directly or indirectly involved in reducing the incidence of harmful alcohol use in the general population.
3.   Suggest one way that you personally could be a "no harmful alcohol use" advocate for each of the two target groups: (1) family; (2) friends.

Chapter Review Test

Multiple Choice: Directions: In the space at the left, write the letter of the choice that best completes each of the following statements.

_____   1.   Differences in drinking patterns between men and women include all of the following EXCEPT: (p. 207)
   a.   Women drink less often
   b.   Women report themselves as heavy drinkers three times as often
   c.   Women suffer fewer problems with drinking
   d.   Women have tended to be more secretive about their drinking

_____   2.   In the college environment, research indicates that the percentage of college students who drink alcohol is: (p. 208))
   a.   30%
   b.   50%
   c.   70%
   d.   90%

_____   3.   A teenager who drinks has what risk of becoming addicted to alcohol as compared to a non-drinking teen. (p. 209)
   a.   2-3 times
   b.   5-7 times
   c.   8-10 times
   d.   12-14 times

_____   4.   College students are motivated to drink because they believe that drinking will: (p. 210)
   a.   increase their interpersonal skills
   b.   allow them to be more socially attractive
   c.   produce feelings of power and reduce tension
   d.   all of the above

_____   5.   Alcohol dependence refers to: (p. 212)
   a.   chronic, excessive use of a drug, such that physical or other personal harm is very likely to occur
   b.   potentially harmful consumption that is not chronic but only an isolated episode
   c.   uncontrolled compulsion to use a drug in spite of physical, emotional, and social problems
   d.   none of the above apply to the definition of alcohol dependence

_____   6.   Alcohol has its most significant health-related impact on which body system? (p.213)
   a.   the central nervous system
   b.   the voluntary muscle system
   c.   the digestive system
   d.   the respiratory system

_____   7. Within minutes after consuming alcohol, the brain changes its functioning capacity in all of the following ways with the EXCEPTION of: (p. 213)
   a. altering judgment
   b. decreasing the time it takes to react
   c. reducing muscle control
   d. reducing concentration

_____   8. This disease results from alcohol destroying liver cells and plugging the liver with fibrous scar tissue which can lead to liver failure and death. (p. 214)
   a. hangover
   b. cirrhosis
   c. pancreatitis
   d. alcohol dementia

_____   9. This syndrome is characterized by a pattern of severe birth defects present in babies born to mothers who drink alcohol during their pregnancy. (p. 214)
   a. fetal alcohol syndrome
   b. Downs syndrome
   c. sudden infant death syndrome
   d. cretinism

_____   10. In recent years, the rate of alcoholism in women has: (p. 207)
   a. decreased
   b. remained the same
   c. increased
   d. exceeded the rate of alcoholism in men

_____   11. A blood alcohol concentration of _____ is considered lethal. (p. 215)
   a. .05
   b. .20
   c. .40
   d. .80

_____   12. The need for higher doses of alcohol in order to reach the same desired effects is called: (p. 218)
   a. addiction
   b. tolerance
   c. physical dependence
   d. psychological dependence

_____   13. A pattern of pathological use of alcohol that results in impaired social or occupational functioning is called: (p. 218)
   a. addiction
   b. tolerance
   c. physical dependence
   d. psychological dependence

_____ 14. An individual who uses alcohol in a manner that causes physical, psychological or social harm to him/herself or others is considered: (p. 218)
   a.   a binge drinker
   b.   a chronic drinker
   c.   a social drinker
   d.   a problem drinker

_____ 15. When the effects of one drug, such as alcohol, are added to the effects of another drug, such as aspirin, the combined impact of the two drugs is greater than would be expected if each drug's effects were simply added together. This phenomenon is referred to as: (p. 226)
   a.   detoxification
   b.   synergism
   c.   molarity
   d.   concentration level

CHAPTER 10
UNDERSTANDING THE DANGERS OF DRUG USE

Chapter Overview

This chapter defines the various types of drugs and how they can affect the user. It specifically examines the impact of illegal drugs and informs the reader how to prevent drug abuse.

What the term "Drug" Means. A drug is any substance that alters the functions of the body whether physically or psychologically and can include *over-the-counter drugs, prescription drugs,* and *dangerous* or *illegal substances* and many other substances such as glue, caffeine, and alcohol. "The Caffeine High" article explains the physiological effects of caffeine. Accompanying this article is a table listing different sources of caffeine.

Who Uses Drugs. Drug use among adolescents or preadolescents often starts with cigarettes and alcohol or *gateway drugs* and can lead to marijuana and other illegal drugs, a progression called *staging.* For various reasons such as peer pressure, relaxation, family influence and alleviating stress, college students are the largest group to use drugs, especially substances that are prohibitive. A table shows the types of drugs and the percentages of college students who use them. *Controlled substances* such as LSD and marijuana, although illegal, are readily available and become inexpensive if they are in high demand. Criminalizing drugs is often considered an unsuccessful approach in curbing drug abuse as shown in the two contrasting professional opinions over whether or not Americans should be allowed to smoke marijuana for medicinal purposes.

From Drug Use to Drug Abuse. *Drug abuse* is the intentional mistreatment of a substance and can lead a person to become *drug dependent;* whose body over time builds up a *tolerance* to the drug; and who often experiences a physical and or *psychological dependence.* In addition, cessation of a drug can cause *withdrawal.* Drugs can attach themselves to *receptor sites* in the brain, affecting a particular organ or tissue by altering, enhancing or diminishing its functions. A chapter table shows the effects of different drugs on the brain. When drugs are combined they can cause *additive, inhibitory or synergistic effects,* which may adversely harm the body.

How Drugs Differ. Drugs can be organized by the methods of consumption, their psychoactive effects, or by the motive of the user. *Stimulants, depressants, hallucinogens, narcotics and cannabis* are all categories used to describe how a person may react to a drug. According to this categorization, detailed examples of illegal drugs are included in the chapter. An accompanying essay examines the growing abuse of steroids among adolescent girls in order to remain thin.

Impact of Drug Abuse. Although drug abuse can cause lasting health damage and even death to the user, it also affects non-users through transmission of the AIDS virus, fetal damage, productivity and safety in the workplace, and drug trafficking.

Treatment Alternatives: The Long Road Back. To treat drug abusers there are *maintenance* and *detoxification programs, therapeutic communities* where people use group therapy over a long period of time, as well as other alternative therapies. Public opinion varies on methods necessary towards solving the drug problem.

Prevention of Drug Abuse: The Skills of Saying "No". Being prepared through the use of personal and social skills such as decision-making and communication even before being confronted with the opportunity to use drugs has been demonstrated as a positive approach to health behavior. Included is a quiz testing how likely you are to take drugs.

There are four **Critical Thinking Questions** interjected throughout the chapter. They discuss: (1) prevention of hard drug use by concentrating on mild drug users; (2) whether or not drug related deaths are a good measurement of drug problems; (3) why high school males continue to use dangerous anabolic steroids; and (4) the effectiveness of the "Say No to Drugs" program on certain demographic groups.

Chapter Focus Questions

1.   What are the differences between over-the-counter drugs, prescription drugs and dangerous or illegal substances?

2.   Who uses drugs and what are the most often used drugs among college students?

3.   What is the concept of staging as it relates to drug use?

4.   What is/are the difference(s) between main effects and side effects of drugs?

5.   What are the dangers of mixing drugs and what is meant by additive, inhibitory and synergistic effects?

6.   How would you group drugs based on: how they are taken, their effects, and the motive of the user?

7.   What is the cost of drug abuse to society?

8.   What are the health risks associated with drug abuse?

9.   According to your text, what are three treatment alternatives for drug abusers?

10.   What specific actions would you suggest can be taken to avoid drug abuse?

Case Study Reflections

Suzy and James are both good students. They study hard the night before a test. Before Suzy retires for the evening she smokes a joint or two to help her relax. The next day she performs poorly on the test. James understands how marijuana can affect the mind adversely and decides not to use the drug.

1. Suzy has progressed from smoking cigarettes to smoking marijuana, but vows that she would never try any other drug. Does the use of marijuana increase the chances to using other drugs? Why or why not?

2. Suzy is not convinced that the joints she smoked affected her test score. What evidence would you suggest to convince her otherwise?

3. On another night, Suzy smokes her usual joint, but instead of feeling relaxed, she becomes high-strung, excessively tense, and then very upset. Why would this reaction occur?

4. Besides "staging," what do you suppose are the reasons for Suzy's drug use? How do you explain James' ability to avoid drug use? What may be the long-term consequences of Suzy's drug habit?

Chapter Activities

A.   Personal Assessment:

Am I "dealing with drugs?" To find out, circle the answer that best applies to you. For this assessment, the term drug means controlled chemicals other than tobacco and alcohol.

		<u>Never</u>		Sometimes		<u>Always</u>
1.	I use drugs for pleasure.	5	4	3	2	1
2.	I use drugs for relaxation.	5	4	3	2	1
3.	I am addicted to drugs.	5	4	3	2	1
4.	Drugs make me feel better.	5	4	3	2	1
5.	I have tried unsuccessfully to quit using drugs.	5	4	3	2	1
6.	When I don't use drugs I suffer from withdrawal symptoms.	5	4	3	2	1
7.	I can refuse a drug when offered.	1	2	3	4	5
8.	I have experienced a drug-related illness.	5	4	3	2	1
9.	I have experienced a drug-related legal consequence.	5	4	3	2	1
10.	I have experienced a drug-related social problem.	5	4	3	2	1
11.	I use drugs for social reasons.	5	4	3	2	1
12.	I have experienced a drug-related blackout.	5	4	3	2	1
13.	I have experienced a drug-related hangover.	5	4	3	2	1
14.	I drive when I am under the influence of drugs.	5	4	3	2	1
15.	I use anabolic steroids.	5	4	3	2	1
16.	I know how to obtain reliable drug-related information, products, and services.	1	2	3	4	5

Conclusion:

1.   Add up your score. The maximum score is 80. The higher the score, the more "drug healthy" you are.

2.   Which area(s) did you score the highest (4 or 5 points)?_____
    _____

3.   Which area(s) did you score the lowest (1 or 2 points)?_____
    _____

4.   What is one change I could make to improve my "drug health" literacy? _____
    _____

B.   Health Enhancement:

1.   You have just inherited a country. What will be your drug laws and consequences?
2.   Evaluate the pros and cons of mandatory drug testing for various occupations (including students).
3.   Should individuals in correction facilities be given any special benefits if they volunteer to participate in drug testing (e.g. HIV testing) programs? Why or why not?
4.   Compare several anti-drug programs in terms of cost and effectiveness.
5.   Design an anti-drug use billboard.

C.   Health Promotion:

1.   List three ways you could be involved in helping to reduce the incidence of harmful drug use in the general population.
2.   List three ways cultural, environmental (physical or social-economic), political, religious, or health care attitudes/actions could be directly or indirectly involved in reducing the incidence of harmful drug use in the general population.
3.   Suggest one way that you personally could be a "no harmful drug use" advocate for each of the two target groups: (1) family; (2) friends.

Chapter Review Test

Multiple Choice: Directions: In the space at the left, write the letter of the choice that best completes each of the following statements.

_____   1. Chemical compounds such as analgesics, cold and flu capsules, laxatives, as well as vitamin and mineral supplements are classified as: (p.233)
   a.   prescription drugs
   b.   illicit drugs
   c.   over-the-counter drugs
   d.   psychoactive drugs

_____   2. In the typical progression of drug use, a person starts with cigarettes, beer or wine and then moves on to marijuana and hard liquor and subsequently to other illicit drugs, a concept called: (p.236)
   a.   compulsive use
   b.   staging
   c.   situational use
   d.   occasional use

_____   3. Researchers have identified several risk factors for drug abuse among older teenagers and young adults, the most consistent and powerful predictor being: (p. 237)
   a.   families
   b.   peer pressure
   c.   psychological variables
   d.   school problems and issues

_____   4. Drugs and/or chemicals like marijuana, heroin and LSD that have been identified through legal review as a threat to an individual or to society are defined as : (p. 238)
   a.   over-the-counter drugs
   b.   prescription drugs
   c.   controlled drugs
   d.   all of the above

_____   5. The intentional misuse of a drug or chemical is called: (p. 240)
   a.   addiction
   b.   withdrawal
   c.   drug misuse
   d.   drug abuse

_____   6. Drugs that cause side effects: (p.240)
   a.   are any effects that are caused by psychoactive drugs
   b.   produce unwanted effects of a drug
   c.   act on specific organs or tissues
   d.   are always negative in nature

_____   7. This term refers to a person's psychological state, including mood or motive: (p. 241)
        a.   host
        b.   environment
        c.   set
        d.   setting

_____   8. When two drugs are present in the system at one time but the effect of one reduces or blocks the effect of the other is referred to as: (p. 241)
        a.   addictive effects
        b.   inhibiting effects
        c.   synergistic effects
        d.   pronounced effects

_____   9. When barbiturates and alcohol are taken together producing an extremely amplified result, the interactive effect is referred to as a(n): (pp. 241-242)
        a.   addictive effect
        b.   inhibitory effect
        c.   synergistic effect
        d.   tolerance

_____   10. A term often used to describe the undesired effects of taking a large amount of a single drug is: (p. 242)
        a.   over-use
        b.   overdose
        c.   misuse
        d.   dosage effect

_____   11. Using this form of drug administration, chemicals produce vapors resulting in psychoactive effects. (pp. 242-243)
        a.   smoked
        b.   inhaled
        c.   swallowed
        d.   ingested

_____   12. The stimulant crack is considered a purified form of this drug producing a rapid and intense reaction: (p. 243)
        a.   opium
        b.   LSD
        c.   barbiturates
        d.   cocaine

_____   13. Amphetamines are stimulants that speed up which system in the body? (p.243)
        a.   respiratory system
        b.   muscular system
        c.   central nervous system
        d.   circulatory system

_____   14. Narcotics act as an analgesic (relieving pain) on the: (p.244)
   a. respiratory system
   b. muscular system
   c. digestive system
   d. central nervous system

_____   15. Which of the following are powerful derivatives from male hormones that produce muscle
        growth and can change health and behavior? (p. 244)
   a. marijuana
   b. anabolic steroids
   c. antihistamines
   d. cocaine

CHAPTER 11
RECOGNIZING VIOLENT BEHAVIOR

Chapter Overview

Living in an environment of violence jeopardizes a person's quality of life, but there are solutions for the individual, such as learning to recognize potential dangerous situations, and using the conflict resolution method. The chapter also outlines becoming an unbiased mediator to prevent other people's conflicts from erupting into violence. Violence is described as any intentional assault which causes harm to persons or property. The chapter argues that violent behavior, in any form, is both a public and private health problem.

Who Commits Acts of Violence? Generalities can be made over who is most likely to commit a violent act. Most offenders tend to be unemployed, users of illicit drugs, with little education, and were often abused as children. Although the majority of perpetrators are young male Caucasians, the percentages of criminal arrests for black men is higher than for white men.

Who is At Risk of Being Assaulted? Except in instances of personal larceny and rape, more men are victims of violent crime than women. African Americans, the elderly, homosexuals, and people of lower income are groups that experience high instances of violent crimes. Almost half of all victims are acquainted with their assailants. For percentages of crime victims, the text contains a table rating amounts by various demographic criteria.

When and Where Crime Takes Place. Because commonalities are also found in the time and place a crime may occur, listed are qualified tips to safeguard your home, your car and yourself to avoid becoming a victim. The more urban the area, the more likely a crime is to take place. Homes are usually robbed during the day, while commercial property is more at risk at night. The weekend, especially Saturday night, has more violent crimes occurring, such as homicide and rape, than during the week. Again, people living in low-income neighborhoods experience more violent crime.

Homicide: Dying in America. Homicide rates in America are high, having risen dramatically from 1985 to 1993. In the text a table shows that homicide rates for minorities are usually higher than the general population, with black males at greatest risk. A comparison of different countries' gun control policies, the amount of gun related homicides and the number of households with guns shows the United States leads in overall firearm possession and gun homicides. America's high homicide rates are also associated with illicit drug dealing and the abusive consumption of illegal drugs and alcohol. Some research suggests that there is a possible link between aggressive behavior and violent acts viewed on television.

Violence at Home and On the Job. The crime of domestic battering is found in forms of *physical abuse* as well as *psychological abuse* and legally includes spouses, non-marital partners, and dates. Although men can be victims of domestic abuse, a graph shows a rise in women who are victims of physical abuse by men. Domestic abuse covers all demographic areas and its rates are presumed to be higher than what is reported because its victims are often silent about their abuse. Listed are questions to ask yourself if trying to detect whether there is abuse in a relationship of your own or someone close to you. Abuse of power is also found in the form of *sexual harassment*, and may lead to forms of violence as evidenced in an article suggesting that harassing e-mails should be included under the domain of stalking laws.

When Children Get Hurt. Child abuse is not only physical battering but is also categorized by emotional abuse, physical neglect, and sexual abuse. Reporting suspected child abuse is a citizen's legal responsibility in many states. Indications of when to suspect child abuse are therefore depicted in the chapter.

The Crime of Rape. Rapists usually know the victim and commit rape out of a need to exert control or to dominate someone else, not because of sexual desire. A table shows the rates of common circumstances surrounding instances of rape. *Acquaintance rape*, such as *date rape* and *marital rape,* constitute the majority of rape crimes, where the victim knows the attacker. Often victims of rape experience what is known as *rape trauma syndrome* which includes immediate feelings of confusion, fear and helplessness later followed by denial and a withdrawing from family and friends. After this period the victim often experiences those same feelings of helplessness and anger that they had in the beginning.

There are three **Critical Thinking Questions** interjected throughout the chapter. They discuss: (1) the possibilities of banning handguns in America; (2) why the rate of women abused by their partners is rising; and (3) whether or not a legal differentiation should exist between date rape and stranger rape.

Chapter Focus Questions

1. How is violent behavior a threat to personal health as well as a threat to the health of the general public?

2. How would you describe the common criminal; that is, the person who commits acts of violence?

3. Who is at risk of being a victim; that is a person who experiences violent crime?

4. It is said that crime does not take place in random fashion. When and where does violent crime usually take place?

5. To what extent are the availability of handguns, television and drugs factors in violent crime?

6. What are some examples of violent behavior found in the home or on the job?

7. What is the prevalence of abuse carried out against women in the United States?

8. What is the difference between physical abuse and physical neglect?

9. How might one describe an abusive relationship?

10. In what way(s) is/are acquaintance rape similar to date rape?

Case Study Reflections

Faye and LaVerne moved to the city after graduating from college. Faye's fear of crime associated with city-living severely diminishes her sense of security and safety. LaVerne, meanwhile, recognizes the danger, takes steps to avoid the danger and experiences the full life a city can provide.

1.   Are Faye's fears real? Is she more at risk in the city than in her rural hometown? Why?

2.   Both Fay and LaVerne each take measures to insure their safety. Whose measures of prevention are better? Why? Does Faye's behavior preclude her from violent crime? Why?

3.   What are the problems, both psychologically and logically, with seeing everyone "as a possible mugger, rapist or robber?"

4.   Before Faye moves back home, a friend of hers suggests she carry a handgun for protection. Why is this not the answer to her problems? What does it say about the culture in which Faye lives?

Chapter Activities

A.   **Personal Assessment:**
     Am I associated with violent behavior? To find out, circle the answer that best applies to you.

		Never		Sometimes		Always
1.	I have a gun in my home.	1	2	3	4	5
2.	I frequently use alcohol or other drugs.	1	2	3	4	5
3.	I have seen domestic violence to others in my family.	1	2	3	4	5
4.	I have been a victim of domestic physical abuse.	1	2	3	4	5
5.	I have been a victim of psychological abuse.	1	2	3	4	5
6.	I have been a victim of sexual abuse or violence.	1	2	3	4	5
7.	I have been a victim of emotional abuse.	1	2	3	4	5
8.	I have been a victim of physical neglect.	1	2	3	4	5
9.	I have been a victim of acquaintance or date rape.	1	2	3	4	5
10.	I know how to access assistance in cases of abuse or violence.	5	4	3	2	1
11.	I know how to obtain reliable violence-related information, products, and services.	5	4	3	2	1

Conclusion:

1.   Add up your score. The maximum score is 55. The higher the score, the higher your "violence and abuse" risk.

2.   Which area(s) did you score the highest (4 or 5 points) ?_____
_____

3.   Which area(s) did you score the lowest (1 or 2 points)?_____
_____

4.   What is one change I could make to improve my "violence reduction" literacy?_____
_____

B.   Health Enhancement:

1.   Develop an evaluation form and monitor several popular TV programs for situations involving violence. Summarize your findings and report to class.
2.   Develop a community resource directory of information, products, and services related to violence prevention.
3.   Generate a list of the places where you believe metal detectors should be installed. Compare your list with other students' lists.
4.   Develop a violence prevention flyer to be distributed in your community.

C.   Health Promotion:

1.   List three ways you could be involved in helping to reduce the incidence of violence in the general population.
2.   List three ways cultural, environmental (physical or social-economic), political, religious, or health care attitudes/actions could be directly or indirectly involved in reducing the incidence of violence in the general population.
3.   Suggest one way that you personally could be a "no violence" advocate for each of the two target groups: (1) family; (2) friends.

Chapter Review Test

Multiple Choice: Directions: In the space at the left, write the letter of the choice that best completes each of the following statements.

_____   1.   Based on the Federal Bureau of Investigation's Uniform Crime Report, violent crimes tend to be committed by: (p. 265)
   a.   young men
   b.   offenders who were abused as children
   c.   offenders who use alcohol and other drugs
   d.   all of the above

_____   2.   Which of the following traits or characteristics do victims of violent crimes share? (pp. 266-267)
   a.   The lower the income, the greater a person is at risk for being a victim.
   b.   The elderly are a vulnerable target for crime.
   c.   Many violent crimes are committed by acquaintances and friends.
   d.   All of the above are true.

_____   3.   More crime takes place in all BUT which of the following cases? (p. 267)
   a.   low-income neighborhoods more than affluent neighborhoods
   b.   rural areas more than in suburbs
   c.   the beginning of the work week (e.g. Monday/Tuesday) more than the weekend
   d.   in the evenings when customers and employees are not likely to be around

_____   4.   Which of the following is the most frequently cited reason offenders give for murder? (p. 269)
   a.   threatened or actual physical abuse had occurred just before the incident
   b.   alcohol and/or drug use
   c.   jealousy, money, or other general stresses of living
   d.   accidental

_____   5.   Deaths as a result of gunshot wounds are most prevalently associated with: (p. 269)
   a.   hunting accidents
   b.   suicides and homicides
   c.   unintentional injuries
   d.   family arguments

_____   6.   Which of the following factors have been linked to violent behavior? (p. 269)
   a.   influence of drugs
   b.   availability of handguns
   c.   viewing violence on TV
   d.   all of the above

_____   7. The phase "violence knows no boundaries" implies: (p. 273)
        a. it crosses socio-economic levels
        b. it occurs among people of all races and religion
        c. it happens in rural and urban areas
        d. all of the above

_____   8. A range of abusive behaviors perpetrated by one member of the family against another, or one "partner" against another is called: (p. 273)
        a. sexual assault
        b. domestic violence
        c. battery
        d. sexual abuse

_____   9. A form of verbal battery which may require the abused person to perform demanding, demeaning and unreasonable tasks is called: (p.274)
        a. physical abuse
        b. psychological abuse
        c. social abuse
        d. sexual abuse

_____   10. Which of the following is NOT a characteristic trait found in abused women? (p. 274)
        a. tend to be submissive
        b. lack in self-confidence
        c. need security and a strong male figure
        d. well educated

_____   11. Which of the following are usually included in general definitions of neglect? (p. 276)
        a. acts of shaking, beating
        b. aggressive behaviors of the child
        c. demeaning comments and put downs
        d. acts of omission

_____   12. Which form of child abuse is exemplified when a child is deprived of the basic necessities of life such as food, clothing and medical care? (p. 276)
        a. emotional abuse
        b. physical neglect
        c. physical abuse
        d. sexual abuse

_____   13. The typical perpetrator of sexual abuse is: (p. 277)
        a. a stranger the victim does not know
        b. a person the child knows
        c. an elderly man who is a pervert
        d. a disabled person who is impotent

_____ 14. Sexual harassment is a criminal offense involving: (p. 278)
   a.   the abuse of power
   b.   personal problems of inadequacy
   c.   a person who is sexually unfulfilled
   d.   women who feel the need for being dominated

_____ 15. Forced sexual intercourse between individuals who know each other is known as: (p. 283)
   a.   sexual assault
   b.   sexual abuse
   c.   acquaintance rape
   d.   sexual harassment

CHAPTER 12
PREVENTING UNINTENTIONAL INJURIES

Chapter Overview

Unintentional injuries, often with serious and lasting disabilities, occur to millions of Americans each year and are the leading cause of death for people ages 15-25. This chapter focuses on what factors put people at risk for injuries and provides suggestions on how to take preventative action to avoid injury.

Accidents and Unintentional Injuries: Cause and Effect. An *accident* is an unintended occurrence that may cause *unintentional injuries*. Usually when these injuries occur, one of the people involved in the accident is careless, lacks specific skills, is unaware, is impaired by substances, or is engaging in risk-taking behavior. People at risk for unintentional injuries tend to be men, lower-income groups, and people living in rural areas. Specific occupations where fatal injuries are most likely to occur is examined in a graph that also includes a list of occupations where fatal injuries were intentional. Not only are these injuries a public health problem, they are a heavy financial burden on society. In the text, a pie chart estimates all costs due to unintentional injuries.

Safety on the Road. Half of all fatal unintentional injuries are the result of motor vehicle accidents, yet there has been a gradual decrease in fatalities throughout the years, primarily as a result of increased seat belt use, air bags and by raising the drinking age to 21. A graph showing how the increased use of seat belts coincided with the lowering of motor vehicle crash deaths further testifies to the success of seat belts to prevent severe injuries and death. Motorcycle injuries tend to be quite severe, often resulting from accidents where the driver was speeding, was not wearing a helmet, had poor skills in operating the cycle and/or had consumed high levels of alcohol. When motorcyclists wear helmets, it greatly increases their chances of surviving an accident An accompanying article shows how to buy the proper helmet for bicycle and motorcycle riders.

Recreational Safety. Severe brain injuries and death can also be prevented when bicyclists wear helmets. Alcohol is a contributing factor in both bicycle and water related injuries including boating accidents, drowning, and diving catastrophes. When young people die from drowning, usually it is the result of *hypothermia*, the loss of body heat, exacerbated when alcohol is present in the bloodstream. Irresponsible divers are often at risk for accidents, the most severe of their non-fatal injuries being *quadriplegia*.

Safety at Home. Falls are one of the most common causes of injuries in the home, with children and the elderly the two most likely groups to harm themselves from a fall. Fires, usually caused by unattended cigarettes, can cause severe burns, damage from smoke inhalation and death. Since the advent of smoke detectors, fire injuries and death have been greatly reduced. Burns can also be attributed to water heaters whose heat levels are set too high and can surprise a person when they expose their skin to running water. Children, being highly susceptible to unintentional burns, are the mot likely group to be burned while handling fireworks. Legislation has helped to prevent many unintentional injuries that occur to children in the home by regulating the sale of fireworks and requiring *child-resistant packaging* of prescription medicines. Although this packaging has protected many children from being poisoned, children are still at risk for ingesting a number of dangerous substances that are left within their reach at home.

Healthskills: Prevention of Unintentional Injuries. Governmental agencies have been established in the interest of public safety to monitor manufacturers, distributors, retailers, and the workplace. The intent here is to regulate the public sector in order to reduce and prevent injuries. However, the responsibility also lies in part with the individual who should create a safe home environment; drive cautiously; wear safety equipment such as helmets, seat-belts, reflective clothing and life jackets; install smoke detectors; keep dangerous chemicals hidden from children; as well as use many other preventative strategies. Learning how to quickly and properly respond in an emergency situation is also critical in preventing unintentional injuries. Some qualified guidelines to follow are: to first try and protect yourself from harm; do not move an injured person unless absolutely necessary; keep victims warm; ask questions from witnesses and victims about the accident and certain important medical information; call 911 or flag down help; administer CPR if possible; and try to control bleeding.

There are four **Critical Thinking Questions** within the chapter. They examine: (1) the reluctance of some Americans to use seat belts, regardless of seat belt's proven safety results; (2) the potential dangers to children from air bags; (3) the ubiquitous use of alcohol in cases of unintentional injuries; and (4) the difficulties in completely preventing injuries by means of instruction in school.

Chapter Focus Questions

1.   How would you differentiate between an accident and an unintentional injury?

2.   How do accidents lead to unintentional injuries?

3.   How would you describe a person who is "at risk" for an unintentional injury?

4.   What is the cost, both monetary and in terms of quality of life, of unintentional injuries to society?

5.   Why are motor vehicle crashes considered the primary cause of unintentional injuries in the United States?

6.   In what ways are seat belts, child safety seats and air bags critical to the reduction of automobile-related injuries?

7.   In what way does alcohol consumption enhance the potential of encountering an unintentional injury?

8.   What recreational activities are sources of unintentional injury?

9.   What are the primary causes of unintentional injuries that occur in the home?

10. What steps are necessary in being prepared to respond when an injury occurs?

Case Study Reflections

In the beginning of chapter 12, Nancy and her friend are hit by a drunk driver. Because seat belts were used and airbags worked appropriately, the two girls escape serious injury. The other driver is fortunate to escape with her life since she was not wearing a seat belt.

1.   Since the drunk driver could still walk a straight line, she thought it was okay for her to drive home. Was this test for sobriety enough to demonstrate a stupor state? Why/why not? How could she have recognized more clearly that she wasn't able to drive after having consumed alcohol?

2.   Another reason the drunk driver thought she could drive herself home was that her house was only a few miles away. Why was this still not a good reason for her to drive?

3.   Nancy and her friend always wear their seat belts. The other driver hardly ever does. What other habits are involved in driver safety?

4.   Might this one incident be enough to change the driving habits of the drunk driver? Why or why not?

Chapter Activities

A.   **Personal Assessment:**
Am I "preventing unintentional injuries?" To find out, circle the answer that best applies to you.

		Never		Sometimes		Always
1.	I live in a rural area.	1	2	3	4	5
2.	I live in a poor urban or rural area.	1	2	3	4	5
3.	I have a high-risk job.	1	2	3	4	5
4.	I use alcohol or other drugs.	1	2	3	4	5
5.	I get adequate sleep.	5	4	3	2	1
6.	I wear seat belts.	5	4	3	2	1
7.	When driving, I exceed the speed limit.	1	2	3	4	5
8.	I wear a helmet when riding on a motorcycle.	5	4	3	2	1
9.	I play contact sports.	1	2	3	4	5
10.	I tend to ignore water-safety rules.	1	2	3	4	5
11.	My residence has hazards (e.g. lighting, electrical, handrails, poisons).	1	2	3	4	5
12.	I smoke when I am tired.	1	2	3	4	5
13.	My residence has smoke, fire, and carbon monoxide detectors.	5	4	3	2	1
14.	I practice a fire-escape plan.	5	4	3	2	1
15.	I know how to obtain reliable injury-related information, products, and services.	5	4	3	2	1

Conclusion:
1.   Add up your score. The maximum score is 75. The lower the score, the lower your risk for unintentional injury.

2.   Which area(s) did you score the highest (4 or 5 points)?_____
_____

3.   Which area(s) did you score the lowest (1 or 2 points)?_____
_____

4.   What is one change I could make to improve my "unintentional injury" literacy?_____
_____

B.   Health Enhancement:

1.   Create a puppet show demonstrating how to reduce the risk of unintentional injury. Perform for the class.
2.   Generate a "new law" designed to reduce the risk of unintentional injury. Have the class critique your new law for feasibility.
3.   Write a children's story with a major theme of preventing unintentional injuries.
4.   Invent a "safety" device.

C.   Health Promotion:

1.   List three ways you could be involved in helping to reduce the incidence of unintentional injuries in the general population.
2.   List three ways cultural, environmental (physical or social-economic), political, religious, or health care attitudes/actions could be directly or indirectly involved in reducing the incidence of unintentional injuries in the general population.
3.   Suggest one way that you personally could be a "no unintentional injury" advocate for each of the two target groups: (1) family; (2) friends.

Chapter Review Test

Multiple Choice: Directions: In the space at the left, write the letter of the choice that best completes each of the following statements:

_____   1. Which of the following is considered to be the leading cause of death among college age students? (p. 290)
  a. homicides
  b. suicides
  c. unintentional injuries
  d. cancer

_____   2. Accidents which are random, uncontrolled acts of fate over which there is little control, or a result of carelessness or ignorance are known as: (p. 290)
  a. homicides
  b. suicides
  c. unintentional injuries
  d. intentional injuries

_____   3. Which of the following factors places people at increased risk of injury? (pp. 292-293)
  a. gender and age
  b. environment
  c. certain occupations
  d. all of the above

_____   4. Studies show that motor vehicle accidents in which alcohol plays a role are: (p. 291)
  a. the number one cause of preventable traffic fatalities
  b. less severe than other crashes
  c. less fatal than other crashes
  d. the fifth leading cause of death for all population groups

_____   5. Which of the following injuries is the result of an environmental factor? (p. 292)
  a. attempted suicide
  b. preventable traffic accident
  c. earthquake or tornado
  d. fall from rock climbing

_____   6. Which of the following population groups accounts for the safest time period for reduced injury rates? (p. 292)
  a. individuals between birth and 5 years of age
  b. individuals between 5-16 years of age
  c. individuals between 15-24 years of age
  d. individuals between 20-40 years of age

_____ 7. Which of the following population groups accounts for the largest percentage of unintentional injuries? (p. 292)
   a. men of all ages
   b. women of all ages
   c. teenagers between the ages of 13-19
   d. elderly citizens over 65 years of age

_____ 8. Which of the following ethnic groups has the highest death rates from unintentional injuries? (p. 292)
   a. African Americans
   b. Caucasians
   c. Asians
   d. Native Americans

_____ 9. On-the-job fatalities are primarily associated with: (p. 293)
   a. falls
   b. electrocutions
   c. motor vehicle accidents
   d. drug use

_____ 10. Only one other cause of premature death exceeds unintentional injuries in incidence among all age groups. That cause is: (p. 293)
   a. cancer
   b. heart disease
   c. homicide
   d. infant mortality

_____ 11. Motor vehicle accidents account for what percent of all unintentional injuries in the U.S.? (p. 296)
   a. one-fourth
   b. one-third
   c. half
   d. two-thirds

_____ 12. Currently, how many states require that at least the people in the front seat of a motorized vehicle use seat belts? (p. 296)
   a. all 50 states
   b. all but two states
   c. only 10 percent
   d. less than one-half

_____ 13. The leading cause of motorcycle injuries is: (p. 300)
   a. not wearing a helmet
   b. alcohol and drugs
   c. not obeying traffic regulations
   d. lack of operator skill

_____   14. Most deaths due to drowning in young adults are: (p. 302)
   a.   alcohol-related
   b.   hypothermia-related
   c.   both a and b
   d.   neither of the two

_____   15. What population group is most at risk for fatal falls? (p. 304)
   a.   men
   b.   women
   c.   small children
   d.   the elderly

CHAPTER 13
REDUCING THE RISK OF CHRONIC DISEASE

Chapter Overview

Chronic diseases develop over a long period of time and are a serious health problem that often leads to eventual death for many Americans, especially African Americans whose percentages of chronic disease are the highest when compared with all other Americans. The quality of life for sufferers is hampered as a result of these debilitating chronic diseases, yet health measures can be taken to alleviate symptoms, prevent diseases and even reverse their effects.

Characteristics of Chronic Illness. A *chronic illness* usually lasts for a long time, causes disability, requires some form of treatment, grows either increasingly better or progressively worse, and is different from an infectious disease in that it is not often communicable. Chronic diseases may result from a genetic predisposition, and/or environmental and behavioral circumstances. Often they take a progressively long time to develop and a long time to treat. A chronic disease is not always apparent in the beginning. During the *asymptomatic period* there are no outward signs of the disease. These appear during the *symptomatic period* when a trained physician can determine the *diagnosis* so a patient may begin treatment. Early detection is the most important way to deter major damage from the disease and it is important for the individual to monitor and regulate certain aspects of their life in order to prevent and/or detect possible disease. Included in the text is a list of common chronic diseases accompanied with their risk factors, symptoms and method of treatment.

From the Heart: Cardiovascular Disease are diseases of the heart and blood vessels. They are the number one cause of death in America, even though the actual rate of deaths from heart disease has dropped in the past 20 years. African Americans are uniquely more at risk for developing heart disease than other Americans. Based on the leading causes of death the text lists the rates of mortality for black American women compared to white American women. Many risk factors for developing heart disease are a result of lifestyle, with smoking the number one factor followed by hypertension (high blood pressure), obesity, diabetes, high cholesterol diets, and poor physical fitness. Heredity is also a factor. An ECG or *electrocardiogram*, is used to detect heart abnormalities that may indicate disease. Cardiovascular diseases range from atherosclerosis (hardening of the arteries) which often causes a *myocardial infarction* (a heart attack), to *angina pectoris*, which temporarily halts blood flow to the heart, *arrhythmia* which is irregular beatings of the heart, *stroke* and *hypertension*. Treatments for heart disease include medication, surgery for clogged arteries, heart transplants, and preventative measures such as exercise and a low-fat diet.

The Big C: Cancer. Although genetics play a part in who gets cancer, a healthy lifestyle increase the chances of not developing cancer. How cancer begins is still unknown, but healthy cells develop into abnormal cancer cells which form into a tumor, believed to occur by the body's exposure to carcinogens. The danger of cancer tumors is that they *metastasize* if left untreated, by the spreading of diseased cells from the place of origin throughout the rest of the body. Smoking, excessive radiation, alcohol abuse, certain foods, lengthy exposure to the sun, especially for fair-skinned people, and toxic chemicals are all believed to contribute to the development of different cancers. The most common cancers are lung, breast, prostate, skin, colon and leukemia. The best way to combat cancer is early detection through pap smears, mammograms, prostate blood tests, self-exams and other screenings. Treatment for cancers include various types of surgery, radiation, chemotherapy and mind-body treatments (considered a psychosomatic approach).

Smile Please: Dental Disease. Widespread, but luckily not life-threatening, are dental diseases. The two categories of dental disease include: *periodontal disease* (gum disease) which results from plaque bacteria that form on the gums, ultimately weakening the gum's ability to support the teeth; and *dental caries* or tooth decay that occurs when plaque builds up on the teeth and forms a cavity. The best prevention is regular brushing with fluoride toothpaste, flossing and professional removal of tartar.

Living with Chronic Disease. One of the side-effects of a chronic disease is the change in a person's psychological well-being as they deal with the difficulties of adjusting to painful symptoms, treatments and disabilities that often change their style of life.

There are four **Critical Thinking Questions** within the text that discuss: (1) what new chronic disease may arise to cause death if today's common diseases were cured; (2) the connection between cholesterol screening and prevention of heart disease; (3) how to educate people about the dangers of artificial light exposure; and (4) the connections between dental disease and other more serious chronic diseases in terms of prevention strategies.

Chapter Focus Questions

1. How would you differentiate between chronic illness and infectious illness?

2. What is meant by the natural history of a chronic illness, including the asymptomatic and symptomatic periods?

3. What lifestyle choices are related to the occurrence of chronic illness?

4. What are the risk factors associated with cardiovascular disease?

5. What are the symptoms and treatment modalities for cardiovascular disease?

6. What are the behavioral risk factors associated with cancer?

7. What are the prevalency rates for the following cancers: lung, breast, cervical, prostate, and stomach?

8. How important is early detection of cancer and what are several screening procedures that can lead to early detection?

9. In terms of severity, how is dental disease compared with more life-threatening forms of chronic illness?

10. In what ways do psychological support and pain management help individuals who have a chronic illness?

Case Study Reflections

Louise and Mariana both detect lumps in their breasts at a relatively early stage. Louise tries to wish the lump away until it becomes dangerously large. Mariana seeks treatment right away. Because of her response, Mariana's breast cancer is treated with minimal risk to her life.

1.   What health habits should Louise and Mariana have been practicing to detect breast cancer? Given that both women survive, how important is early detection and treatment in chronic illness?

2.   Both women have twenty-year-old daughters. What influence do their mothers' illnesses have on their lives? Louise's daughter has been diagnosed to have both genes BRCA1 and BRCA2. What is the connection between these two genes and cancer?

3.   Name several ways Louise and Mariana's daughters can reduce their risk for breast cancer.

4.   What if any psychological adjustments did Louise and Mariana have to make during their cancer illness? Is there any danger in their cancer reappearing?

Chapter Activities

A. **Personal Assessment:**
Do I "reduce my risk of chronic disease"? To find out, circle the answer that best applies to you.

		Never		Sometimes		Always
1.	My lifestyle choices increase my risk of chronic disease.	1	2	3	4	5
2.	I take advantage of available health screening techniques that will affect my risk of chronic disease.	5	4	3	2	1
3.	My genetic predisposition will increase my risk of chronic disease.	1	2	3	4	5
4.	My gender will affect my risk of chronic disease.	1	2	3	4	5
5.	My age will affect my risk of chronic disease.	1	2	3	4	5
6.	I smoke.	1	2	3	4	5
7.	I have hypertension which will affect my risk of chronic disease.	1	2	3	4	5
8.	I have elevated cholesterol which will affect my risk of chronic disease.	1	2	3	4	5
9.	I have elevated iron in my blood.	1	2	3	4	5
10.	I am overweight.	1	2	3	4	5
11.	Adult-onset diabetes will affect my risk of chronic disease.	1	2	3	4	5
12.	I have a sedentary lifestyle.	1	2	3	4	5
13.	I have repeated exposure to sunlight over a long period of time.	1	2	3	4	5
14.	I consume excessive amounts of alcohol.	1	2	3	4	5
15.	I am exposed to toxic fumes, gasses, airborne particles, and liquids.	1	2	3	4	5

		Never		Sometimes		Always
16.	I am exposed to asbestos, vinyl chloride.	1	2	3	4	5
17.	I get dental check-ups.	5	4	3	2	1
18.	I know how to obtain reliable chronic disease-related information, products, and services.	5	4	3	2	1

Conclusion:

1.   Add up your score. The maximum score is 90. The higher the score, the more chronic disease risk you have.

2.   Which area(s) did you score the highest (4 or 5 points)?_____
_____

3.   Which area(s) did you score the lowest (1 or 2 points)?_____
_____

4.   What is one change I could make to lower my chronic disease risk?_____
_____

B.   Health Enhancement:

1.   Develop (invent) a "quackery" or fraudulent product designed to cure one or more chronic conditions. Give a sales pitch and try to "sell" it to the class.
2.   Cigarette smoking speeds up the heart. Exercise speeds up the heart. Therefore you can do either to "exercise and strengthen" your heart. Critique this conclusion.
3.   Rank and justify the leading risk factors for cardiovascular disease. Do the same for cancer.
4.   Research the relationship between genetics and chronic diseases.
5.   Develop several "Jeopardy" (the game show) questions about chronic diseases. Challenge your classmates!

C.   Health Promotion:

1.   List three ways you could be involved in helping to reduce the risk of chronic disease in the general population.
2.   List three ways cultural, environmental (physical or social-economic), political, religious, or health care attitudes/actions could be directly or indirectly involved in reducing the risk of chronic disease in the general population.
3.   Suggest one way that you personally could be a "reduce the risk of chronic disease" advocate for each of the two target groups: (1) family; (2) friends.

Chapter Review Test

Multiple Choice: Directions: In the space at the left, write the letter of the choice that best completes each of the following statements:

_____ 1. The rates for chronic conditions such as heart disease and cancer are the highest for what target population group? (p. 317)
a. young children
b. teenagers
c. frequent hospital patients
d. the elderly

_____ 2. Chronic illnesses have all BUT which of the following common characteristics/traits? (p. 318)
a. result in some form of permanence
b. result in some form of disability
c. are progressive in nature
d. require short periods of care

_____ 3. Chronic diseases differ from infections diseases in what way? (p. 318)
a. Chronic diseases are generally contagious.
b. Chronic diseases are mostly a result of inherited factors or lifestyle.
c. Chronic diseases usually develop quickly and last a comparatively brief period.
d. Persons with a chronic disease may recover completely.

_____ 4. In what period of the natural history of a disease are there no outward signs or clinical symptoms? (p. 319)
a. asymptomatic period
b. symptomatic period
c. recovery period
d. post-symptomatic period

_____ 5. Which of the following lifestyle factors is NOT considered a major risk factor for cardiovascular disease? (p. 319)
a. smoking and heavy alcohol consumption
b. poor diet
c. failure to exercise
d. genetic predisposition

_____ 6. Which of the following statements is true regarding cardiovascular diseases? (p. 322)
a. They are less common than cancers.
b. They can all be prevented by changing one's lifestyle.
c. They are the leading cause of death in the United States.
d. The rates are higher for Caucasians then among African Americans.

_____   7. Recent research findings documenting the relationship between estrogen and heart disease
               is: (p. 323)
               a. Premenopausal women frequently have a heart attack.
               b. Women who have a hysterectomy before natural menopause have a reduced risk for
                   cardiovascular disease.
               c. Women who take replacement estrogen after menopause have less coronary disease then
                   women who do not take estrogen.
               d. Premenopausal women are at the same risk for cardiovascular disease as men of the
                   same age.

_____   8. Which of the following lifestyle factors is the single most important risk factor associated
               with heart disease? (p. 324)
               a. smoking
               b. hypertension
               c. elevated cholesterol
               d. overweight

_____   9. This technique employed for screening as well as detecting heart disease makes use of
               electrodes attached to the body which transmit electrical impulses from the heart to a device
               that records them. (p. 325)
               a. electromyopathy
               b. electrocardiogram
               c. cardiogram
               d. biopsy

_____   10. The most common form of hardening of the arteries in which fatty substances are deposited
               on arterial walls is called: (p. 325)
               a. hypertension
               b. tachycardia
               c. atherosclerosis
               d. angina pectoris

_____   11. Feelings of discomfort and/or chest pains occurring as a result of a temporary reduction in
               the blood supply to the heart is called: (p. 326)
               a. angina pectoris
               b. myocardial infarction
               c. stroke
               d. arrhythmia

_____   12. A cerebrovascular accident is also called a(n): (p. 326)
               a. arrhythmia
               b. stroke
               c. myocardial infarction
               d. heart attack

_____   13. The lifestyle behavior that most often results in death from cancer is: (p. 332)
  a.   smoking
  b.   repeated exposure to sunlight
  c.   excessive amounts of alcohol
  d.   certain types of food consumption

_____   14. The most common site of cancer for both men and women is the: (p. 334)
  a.   lung
  b.   skin
  c.   colon or rectum
  d.   bladder

_____   15. In this cancer detecting diagnosis, a physician uses a hollow lighted tube to inspect the rectum and lower colon. (p. 338)
  a.   digital rectal exam
  b.   stool blood test
  c.   proctology exam
  d.   sigmoidoscopy

CHAPTER 14
REDUCING THE RISK OF INFECTIOUS DISEASE

Chapter Overview

A contagious disease is spread by agents, such as viruses or bacteria, from an infected source to persons who were previously not infected. This chapter describes the various infectious diseases, how they are contacted, who is at risk, and how individuals can protect themselves from acquiring a communicable disease.

How Diseases are Spread. A *pathogen,* or microorganism, is the causative agent of disease, that lives in the *reservoir of the pathogen*, either a human or animal carrier. The pathogen leaves this carrier through a *portal of exit*, often a bodily fluid, and moves by some means of *transmission* through an *entry into a new host*. The spread of disease is successful when the new host accepts the pathogen. This acceptance is based upon the *susceptibility of the host*. These six factors make up what is called a *chain of infection* that explains how infectious diseases may spread throughout a community. Diseases are caused by six essential pathogens: bacteria, viruses, protozoa, parasitic worms, fungi and prions. The body can come in contact with a pathogen through the air, direct physical contact, contaminated food and water. Some pathogens exist dormant in the body and can be triggered to produce symptoms by certain changes to the body. Not everyone exposed to pathogens develops a full-blown case of a disease for they may have been exposed to low dosages, the pathogen's virulence may have been weak or the individual had a strong resistance. The body protects itself from disease through *non-specific defense mechanisms* such as membranes, sneezing, *phagocytes* which are defensive white blood cells, *interferon*, a virus reducing chemical, and *inflammation*.

Immunity: The Final Line of Defense. Antibodies are proteins in the body that once exposed to a specific *antigen* (foreign diseased substance), learn how to protect the body from the same disease if exposed to it at a later time. Antibodies are also responsible for both *active immunity* (lifelong resistance to a specific disease), and *passive immunity* (immunity from an outside source). Vaccinations are shots that create immunity from certain diseases. The immune system has diseases of its own including allergies and immune deficiency diseases. The stages an infected person may experience once they have a disease are *incubation* (no symptoms yet evident), the *prodromal stage* (highly contagious stage), the *acute stage* (symptoms most prominent), followed by *convalescence,* and *recovery*.

Common Infectious Diseases. No one is immune from the common cold for there are numerous strains of the cold virus, yet no known cure for any of them. Influenza also has many strains, but annual vaccinations may prevent many cases of infection. Vaccinations also protect against different types of pneumonia, but if infected, antibiotics can be used as a treatment. Tuberculosis once was a fatal disease, yet now can be treated with drugs. Three types of Hepatitis are: Hepatitis A, curable and the least problematic; Hepatitis B, which is more severe and transferred through bodily fluids; and Type C which is spread primarily by blood, with its symptoms being chronic. Other common diseases include mononucleosis, lyme disease, chronic fatigue syndrome, and nosocomial infections, which are acquired from hospitals. Childhood diseases such as measles, mumps and rubella have been greatly reduced through vaccinations. Some research suggests that viruses may be the cause of certain chronic diseases or mental disorders. Even though vaccinations have eradicated many diseases, the numbers of infectious disease cases are on the rise. Because pathogens have an amazing capacity to mutate and persist, new infectious diseases will continue to emerge.

Protection Through Prevention. When the public is well-informed, individuals act responsibly to protect themselves from possible infections. Education is the beginning step to protecting yourself from communicable diseases. Healthy exercise and eating habits, regular vaccinations, and good hygiene are a few responsible actions to maintain. An accompanying article shows that a large number of infectious diseases could be kept from spreading if more people simply washed their hands.

There are five **Critical Thinking Questions** interjected throughout the text. The first questions whether people should still be vaccinated for diseases that have had no reported cases for many years. The second discusses how to insure that people obtain necessary immunizations while the third examines the financial savings that would result if intense campaigns were undertaken to eradicate certain infectious diseases through immunizations. The fourth discusses the dangers to both the individual and society that are associated with the improper use of antibiotics. The last imagines the possible consequences of the HIV virus mutating into an organism that could be easily transmitted through casual contact, like the common cold.

Chapter Focus Questions

1.   How are infectious diseases spread from one person to another?

2.   What are the characteristics of the seven families of pathogens?

3.   What are the body's non-specific and specific defense mechanisms against infection?

4.   In what four ways can pathogens get into a person's body?

5.   How might virulence, dosage and resistance influence the spread of infectious disease?

6.   How does immunity function in the maintenance of good health?

7.   How would you differentiate between active immunity and passive immunity?

8.   How would you describe the progress of a disease once infection has occurred?

9.   What are some common symptoms shared by various infectious diseases?

10.   What actions can an individual take to reduce the risk of acquiring an infectious disease?

Case Study Reflections

Beth and Kim both contract infectious diseases during the school year. Antibiotics have been prescribed for Beth's strep throat, but she fails to take the medication as directed? Consequently she suffers a relapse. Kim, on the other hand, rests long enough to recover completely from the flu before resuming her harried life schedule.

1.   Describe each of the two illnesses at the microscopic level. What is the cause of each illness?

2.   As mentioned above, Beth and Kim treat their respective disease in different ways; one with antibiotics, the other with rest and fluids. How does each prescription for treatment assist the healing process?

3.   Why does Beth's relapse cause her to feel even worse?

4.   Name five ways Beth and Kim can help prevent contracting infections in the future. What level in the "chain of infection" do these preventive measures target?

Chapter Activities

A.   Personal Assessment:
Am I reducing my "risk of infectious disease?" To find out, circle the answer that best applies to you.

		Never		Sometimes		Always
1.	My immunizations are up-to-date.	1	2	3	4	5
2.	I wash my hands after bathroom visits.	1	2	3	4	5
3.	I wash my hands frequently during the winter months.	1	2	3	4	5
4.	My genetic background includes immune deficiency diseases.	5	4	3	2	1
5.	I am at risk of HIV infection.	5	4	3	2	1
6.	I have blood-to-blood contact with others.	5	4	3	2	1
7.	I consider food safety when preparing foods.	1	2	3	4	5
8.	I have good eating habits.	1	2	3	4	5
9.	I have good exercise habits.	1	2	3	4	5
10.	I get plenty of rest.	1	2	3	4	5
11.	I maintain a positive mental attitude.	1	2	3	4	5
12.	I bathe on a regular basis.	1	2	3	4	5
13.	I brush my teeth on a regular basis.	1	2	3	4	5
14.	I treat all minor infections seriously.	1	2	3	4	5
15.	I know how to obtain reliable infectious disease-related information, products, and services.	1	2	3	4	5

Conclusion:

1.   Add up your score. The maximum score is 75. The higher the score, the higher your protection against infectious disease.

2.   Which area(s) did you score the highest (4 or 5 points)?_____
_____

3.   Which area(s) did you score the lowest (2 or 3 points)?_____
_____

4.   What is one change I could make to lower my infectious disease risk?_____
_____

B.   Health Enhancement:

1.   With classmates, generate a list of movies that focused on infectious diseases. Determine if the information in the movie was fictitious, plausible, fact — or some other category.
2.   Create a TV commercial designed to help viewers reduce their risk of infectious disease.
3.   With a couple classmates, perform a "mystery skill" illustrating a risky situation for transmitting an infectious disease to the entire class. After the skit, see if the class can identify the disease by asking questions to the actors. Answers can be only "yes" or "no."
4.   Write (and perform) a ballad focusing on an infectious disease.
5.   Design a pamphlet for new mothers encouraging and informing them of the recommended immunization routine for their newborn baby.

C.   Health Promotion:

1.   List three ways you could be involved in helping to reduce the risk of infectious disease in the general population.
2.   List three ways cultural, environmental (physical or social-economic), political, religious, or health care attitudes/actions could be directly or indirectly involved in reducing the risk of infectious disease in the general population.
3.   Suggest one way that you personally could be a "reduce the risk of infectious disease" advocate for each of the two target groups: (1) family; (2) friends.

Chapter Review Test

Multiple Choice: Directions: In the space at the left, write the letter of the choice that best completes each of the following statements:

_____   1.   A disease-causing agent is called a(n): (p. 353)
a.   pathogen
b.   leukocyte
c.   erythrocyte
d.   T-cell

_____   2.   This disease is an example of a parasitic infection caused by not cooking meat thoroughly. (p. 355)
a.   malaria
b.   amoebic dysentery
c.   trichinosis
d.   rabies

_____   3.   In humans, fungi tend to invade: (p. 355)
a.   internal organs
b.   the surface of the skin
c.   the sensory organs
d.   the reproductive organs

_____   4.   Rickettsial infection is usually transmitted by: (p.355)
a.   allergens
b.   contaminated water
c.   insects
d.   contaminated in the atmosphere

_____   5.   The degree or level of strength of a causative agent is referred to as its: (p. 358)
a.   vector
b.   allergen
c.   antibody
d.   virulence

_____   6.   Which of the following conditions is associated with whether or not a person will get sick? (pp. 357-358)
a.   the virulence or strength of the causative agent
b.   the dosage of the causative agent
c.   the degree of resistance of the individual to infection
d.   all of the above

_____   7. What is the body's first line of defense against disease? (p. 358)
   a. the white blood cells that attack the foreign invaders
   b. the inflammatory response
   c. the skin and mucous membranes
   d. vaccines

_____   8. Phagocytes are: (p. 359)
   a. white blood cells that can digest some foreign substances
   b. vaccines
   c. the parts of a pathogen that link with human cells
   d. inflammatory agents

_____   9. Passive immunity: (p. 359)
   a. inhibits the body's natural immune system
   b. lasts only a few weeks
   c. provides long term protection against a specific disease
   d. causes an inflammatory response

_____   10. Disease where antibodies attack the body's own cells of the immune system are called: (p. 362)
   a. autoimmune diseases
   b. chronic diseases
   c. proto immune diseases
   d. monoimmune diseases

_____   11. The stage of an infectious disease when the organism invades the host is the: (p. 363)
   a. prodromal stage
   b. incubation period
   c. acute stage
   d. convalescence period

_____   12. Hepatitis is a viral infection that causes enlargement and pain of the: (p. 370)
   a. kidneys
   b. colon
   c. liver
   d. gall bladder

_____   13. Hospital-acquired diseases, which are caused mostly by bacteria are called: (p. 371)
   a. social infections
   b. hospice infections
   c. nosocomial infections
   d. prodromal infections

_____   14. The disease caused by tick bites resulting in flu-like symptoms, rash and joint pains is known as: (p.371)
  a. Lyme disease
  b. strep throat
  c. AIDS
  d. hepatitis

_____   15. A condition characterized by neurological disorders and swelling of the brain is known as: (p. 375)
  a. Lyme disease
  b. Reyes syndrome
  c. Legionaires disease
  d. hepatitis

CHAPTER 15
REDUCING THE RISK OF SEXUALLY TRANSMITTED DISEASES

Chapter Overview

Sexually transmitted diseases are a significant health problem, in part because they are difficult to monitor and are easily spread through unsafe sexual practices, usually to people ages 15 through 29. This chapter defines various STDs and explains how to prevent, treat and control them.

What are STDs? Sexually transmitted diseases often go untreated because symptoms may not occur immediately or at all. During the *incubation period* of the disease *asymptomatic carriers,* who are not aware that they have an STD, may unknowingly spread the disease. To best control STDs, there should be a combined effort of prevention and treatment by practicing safe sex, seeking regular medical examinations, informing all sexual partners if infected, and following through with medical treatment. When choosing to have sex, you should communicate with potential partners about the possibilities for STDs, use condoms, get tested beforehand, be aware that certain sexual activities are more risky than others for spreading STDs, and use proper hygiene before and after sex.

Viral Diseases. Most viral STDs can not be cured and although some may go into remission, the disease is always present in the body. *Human immunodeficiency virus (HIV)* is an infection which can evolve into the *acquired immune deficiency syndrome (AIDS)*, destroying the body's natural immunity against disease. Most people who die from AIDS develop an *opportunistic disease* such as Kaposi's sarcoma or invasive cervical cancer, which is the ultimate cause of death. HIV is spread through blood, semen and vaginal fluid, not saliva or casual physical contact. Some treatments, such as *protease inhibitors* which slow the replication process of infected cells, have forestalled the progression of the disease, but there still is no cure for AIDS. Genital warts are caused by the *human papilloma virus,* in which there is no test that can confirm the existence of the virus in asymptomatic carriers. There is also no known cure for genital warts. Although, *Hepatitis B* can be sexually transmitted, there are other ways of contacting the disease. Prevention with a vaccine is successful for those people who feel they may be at risk. *Genital herpes,* which manifests itself with painful blisters and sores, is also an incurable viral STD, and can affect children born to mothers of the disease.

Bacterial Diseases. Bacterial STDs can be cured. If diagnosed early enough, lasting damage to the body can be prevented. *Chlamydia trachomatis*, is the most widespread STD. It also is easy to cure if caught early on, yet if left untreated, may cause blindness in newborn children, sterility, or lead to *pelvic inflammatory disease (PID)*. *Gonorrhea* has noticeable symptoms in men, yet, usually not in women. This STD may cause urinary problems, sterility, PID, and blindness in newborns. It can be cured with antibiotics, yet there are strains of the disease that resist treatment. *Syphilis*, once a disease that usually meant the infected person would ultimately experience brain damage, loss of muscle control and death, can not be treated with penicillin.

Other STDs include types of *vaginitis.* The two most common forms of vaginitis are: a yeast or fungus infection, treated with over the counter antifungal drugs; and *trichomoniasis*, treated with an antiprotozoal drug. Neither of these cause serious health risks. There are, however, several practical ways to avoid developing these infections. Parasites can be transmitted by sexual contact and show up on the genital area as lice or scabies, and treated with insecticide shampoos and topical creams. For a complete list of types, symptoms, treatments and preventative methods for STDs, the text provides an overview of the common sexually transmitted diseases.

Safer Sex. No amount of safety precautions will completely guarantee against contacting a sexually transmitted disease; however, if people use safer sex practices, their risks are substantially lowered. Preparation before sex, correct condom use, understanding the risks of all types of sexual activity, and getting regular check-ups will decrease the chances of contracting an STD.

There are four **Critical Thinking Questions** within the text. The first discusses the potential risks people take when they believe they are safe from STDs if they are in a monogamous relationship or because they have ceased sexual activity. The second questions whether the public health methods that contributed to the decline of syphilis cases would also help decrease the prevalence of other STDs. The third examines the efficacy of practicing safe or safer sex to prevent STDs, and the fourth questions why people's use of condoms is still low, regardless of a condom's protection against STDs.

Chapter Focus Questions

1. Why are sexually transmitted diseases considered a major public health problem in the United States today?

2. While many STD's can be cured, why is it that these diseases have not been brought under control?

3. What is the significance of asymptomatic carriers to the overall STD epidemic?

4. How are most STD's spread?

5. What are the primary prevention measures that reduce the potential of contracting an STD?

6. What are the differences between the viral STD's such as HIV/AIDS, hepatitis B, human papilloma virus and genital herpes?

7. What are the differences between the bacterial STD's such as chlamydia, gonorrhea and syphilis?

8. What are the differences between vaginitis, and pubic lice and scabies?

9. What does the concept of "safer sex" mean?

10. At what point in time when the symptoms of STD's appear should one seek an STD examination from a physician?

Case Study Reflections

John and Leon were both sexually active. John normally practiced safe sex to avoid fathering a child, but he failed to do so all the time and consequently contracted herpes. Leon's knowledge about the AIDS virus led him to practice safe sex in all circumstances.

1. Why did John not think himself susceptible to STDs? After referring to the chapter and especially to figure 15.1, "The Cycle of STD Transmission," why is this a mistaken assumption?

2. When John didn't buy a condom before having sex he would rationalize by saying, "Condom's aren't 100 percent sure anyway." Is his statement true? How does the quote apply to John's sexual life? How does the statement relate to John's risk to STDs?

3. Compare John's motivation for using a condom to Leon's motivation. How is one's motivation related to one's behavior?

4. After several months of dating, Leon is considering proposing, but Inge suddenly develops the symptoms of a serious STD. How might the relationship be affected as a consequence of this diagnosis? How would you react if you were Leon?

Chapter Activities

A.   Personal Assessment:

Am I reducing my risk of sexually transmitted diseases? To find out, circle the answer that best applies to you.

		Never		Sometimes		Always
1.	I know the signs and symptoms of the common STDs.	1	2	3	4	5
2.	I have multiple sex partners.	5	4	3	2	1
3.	I participate in activities that allow the movement of pathogens from one individual to me through the genitalia or other tissue such as the mouth or anus.	5	4	3	2	1
4.	I know the sexual history of my sexual partners.	1	2	3	4	5
5.	I abstain from sexual contact.	1	2	3	4	5
6.	Prophylactics (male or female) containing nonoxymol-9 are used during sexual contact.	1	2	3	4	5
7.	My behavior places me at risk of STD infection.	5	4	3	2	1
8.	My partner(s) place me at risk of STD infection.	5	4	3	2	1
9.	I can communicate my feelings about safer sex to my current or potential partner.	1	2	3	4	5
10.	I know how to access current information about STDs.	1	2	3	4	5
11.	I know how to access products and services about STDs.	1	2	3	4	5
12.	I visually examine my partner's genitals prior to engaging in sexual intercourse.	1	2	3	4	5
13.	I participate in sexual activity that often results in tearing of tissues and some bleeding.	5	4	3	2	1
14.	My partner washes his/her genitals with warm soap and water before sexual contact.	1	2	3	4	5

		Never		Sometimes		Always
15.	I wash my genitals with warm soap and water before and after sexual contact.	1	2	3	4	5
16.	I know how to obtain reliable STD-related information, products and services.	1	2	3	4	5

Conclusion:

1. Add up your score. The maximum score is 80. The higher the score, the higher your protection against sexually transmitted diseases.

2. Which area(s) did you score the highest (4 or 5 points)?_____
_____

3. Which area(s) did you score the lowest (1 or 2 points)?_____
_____

4. What is one change I could make to lower my sexually transmitted disease risk?_____
_____

B.   Health Enhancement:

1. With a target audience of high school students, develop a Public Service Announcement (PSA) that is designed to reduce their risk of STDs. Try to have it aired in the community or in some local high schools.
2. Imagine yourself as a parent of a teenager. Role play how you would "teach" your child about STDs.
3. Create a bumper sticker focusing on reducing the risk of STDs.
4. Watch several soap operas. Tabulate the number of times (situations) where an STD could be transmitted. Is there a higher number "shown" on any specific day of the week? Do some soap operas "show" these situations more than others? What other trends are evident?
5. Research the incidence of STDs worldwide. Justify the differences.

C.   Health Promotion:

1. List three ways you could be involved in helping to reduce the risk of sexually transmitted diseases in the general population.
2. List three ways cultural, environmental (physical or social-economic), political, religious, or health care attitudes/actions could be directly or indirectly involved in reducing the risk of sexually transmitted diseases in the general population.
3. Suggest one way that you personally could be a "reduce the risk of sexually transmitted disease" advocate for each of the two target groups: (1) family; (2) friends.

Chapter Review Test

Multiple Choice: Directions: In the space at the left, write the letter of the choice that best completes each of the following statements:

_____   1. The primary risk factor associated with the spread of STDs is: (p. 383)
    a. the birth control pill
    b. the use of alcohol and other drugs
    c. multiple sex partners
    d. reluctance in informing sexual partners

_____   2. Although STDs are caused by a variety of organisms, they all share one common factor: (p. 381)
    a. non-infectious
    b. cure rate is very low
    c. an affinity for the moist, warm genital areas
    d. expensive to treat

_____   3. AIDS is caused by the virus: (p. 386)
    a. herpes simplex
    b. Kaposis sarcoma
    c. human immunodeficiency
    d. human papillomas

_____   4. AIDS is caused by a virus that attacks the: (p. 387)
    a. helper T-cells
    b. red blood cells
    c. respiratory system
    d. circulatory system

_____   5. AIDS is known to be transmitted by all of the following EXCEPT: (pp. 389-390)
    a. direct sexual contact
    b. sharing IV needles
    c. transfusions and infected blood
    d. insects

_____   6. Which of the following is NOT a high risk body fluid for HIV transmission? (p. 389)
    a. blood
    b. saliva or tears
    c. semen
    d. vaginal fluid

_____ 7. Drug therapy, such as protease inhibitors, used to treat people with HIV, appears to: (p. 390)
   a. cure HIV indefinitely
   b. inhibit the replication of HIV
   c. restore normal immune levels
   d. increase the amount of HIV in a person's blood

_____ 8. This virus causes genital warts or small bumps on the genitals. (p. 391)
   a. herpes simplex
   b. Kaposis sarcoma
   c. human immunodeficiency virus
   d. human papillomas virus

_____ 9. Hepatitis B is spread in all of the following ways EXCEPT: (p. 392)
   a. sexual contact
   b. contaminated food
   c. intravenous drug use
   d. body fluids such as blood and semen

_____ 10. Genital herpes, a viral infection causing cold sores or fever blisters is also referred to as: (p. 392)
   a. herpes simplex type 2
   b. pubic lice (crabs)
   c. chlamydia
   d. syphilis

_____ 11. The most prevalent STD in the United States today is: (p. 393)
   a. gonorrhea
   b. syphilis
   c. chlamydia
   d. herpes simplex

_____ 12. The serious complication from chlamydia infection for women is: (p. 393)
   a. pelvic inflammatory disease
   b. vaginitis
   c. yeast infection
   d. pubic lice

_____ 13. Eighty percent of women with gonorrhea are: (p. 394)
   a. middle-aged
   b. in poor health
   c. symptomatic
   d. asymptomatic

_____   14. The main treatment for syphilis since 1947 is: (p. 394)
    a. vaccines
    b. aspirin
    c. AZT
    d. Penicillin

_____   15. Another term for pubic lice is: (p. 399)
    a. genital warts
    b. crabs
    c. spiders
    d. warts

CHAPTER 16
SEXUALITY: DEVELOPING HEALTHY RELATIONSHIPS

Chapter Overview

Healthy sexuality includes the ability to develop positive intimate relationships, to enjoy erotic stimulation, to understand and be at ease with your chosen gender and sex roles, and to make responsible decisions about your own sexuality. This chapter explains different aspects of sexuality and includes an in-depth primer on reproductive anatomy and physiology that illustrates in detail the sexual body.

Points of View About Sexuality. The culture in which you grew up, your religious beliefs or those of your upbringing, your personal experiences and physical makeup and health, all affect your sexual attitudes and practices. Hormones that determine gender and other sexual characteristics such as decreased sex drive and infertility are referred to as *androgens* in men and *estrogens* in women. *Sexual orientation* determines whether people will have a lasting attraction to both sexes (bisexuality), the same sex (homosexuality), or the opposite sex (heterosexuality). Legal and social prejudice still exists for homosexuals and bisexuals, even though research has shown that sexual orientation is not a choice but rather an involuntary condition. Communication is the most important way to help build healthy sexual and intimate relationships.

Love: The Basis of Intimate Relationships. There are three components of love: *intimacy, passion* and *commitment.* Different relationships occur with one or more combinations of these components, but when all three are present in a relationship, it is considered consummate love. The other types may be *romantic love, fatuous love, companionate love, liking, infatuation,* or *empty love.*

Sexual Relationships. The *sex drive* or *libido* is the body's natural, biological desire to engage in sexual activity, usually through physical stimulation of the *erogenous zones* with a partner or by *masturbation.* For arousal, people engage in *foreplay, outercourse* which is stimulation of the genitals, sexual fantasy and other styles of sexual pleasuring.

The Body's Sexual Response. The physiological changes that occur during sexual stimulation are *vasocongenstion,* the increased flow of blood to the sexual organs and other parts of the body, and *myotonia* which describes the spasms, tensions and release of muscles during sex. Two well-known sex therapists, Masters and Johnson, developed a four-stage model to define the physical responses to sexual activity. The four stages are labeled: *excitement, plateau, orgasm,* and *resolution.* Some sex therapists include a fifth stage, *desire,* to preclude the excitement stage.

Sexual Dysfunctions. Some people may experience sexual problems, called dysfunctions, that interfere with their ability to maintain a healthy sexual life. These include *organic* or internal physical problems, external hindrances such as medications or illnesses and psychological obstacles. Dysfunctions that occur to both men and women include *inhibited sexual desire* and sexual addictions. Unique male dysfunctions may be *premature ejaculation* and *impotence.* Women unable to achieve orgasm may be experiencing a condition called *female orgasmic disorder.* Other female dysfunctions include *vaginismus,* the closing of the vagina and *dyspareunia* which causes painful intercourse and usually can be cured with lubricants or increased foreplay. Most sexual dysfunctions should be evaluated by a physician and may be treated with education, therapy or medication.

There are four **Critical Thinking Questions** within the chapter which discuss what types of drugs or new technologies may cause a different sexual revolution in the future: (1) the potential public health problems associated with sexually active teenagers; (2) if violence and prejudice against gays and lesbians are the result of stereotypes and not personal experience; (3) in what ways could the public change its attitudes towards these groups; and (4) the importance of sexual education for young people.

Chapter Focus Questions

1. What collection of qualities make up a person's sexual attitudes, influence a person's sexual behaviors and affect relationships with others?

2. What relationship/connection does gender identity and sex role have to sexuality?

3. What are the differences in sexual practice and attitudes between cultures and between individuals within a particular culture?

4. How do hormones influence sexual development and secondary sex characteristics?

5. What are the differences between the following sexual orientations: heterosexuality, homosexuality and bisexuality?

6. How is it that when verbal and nonverbal languages conflict, miscommunication about sexual desires can result?

7. How might you define love in terms of intimacy, passion and commitment?

8. Is masturbation a form of outercourse or intercourse?

9. How would you describe and compare the four phases of human sexual response; namely excitement, plateau, orgasm and resolution?

10. What sexual dysfunctions occur in both men and women; and which ones occur in men alone and in women alone?

Case Study Reflections

Marisa is in a superficial relationship with Jorge, who is pressuring her to have sex. Because of a lack of intimacy between them, she breaks off her relationship. Alan and Nadia, meanwhile, have an open, trusting relationship in which they both feel comfortable with each other.

1.   After reading the chapter, what "components of love" were present in Jorge and Marisa's relationship? How would you categorize their relationship?

2.   Why is Alan and Nadia's relationship considered a healthy one? What "love components" are present? How would you categorize their relationship?

3.   Communication is positive in any relationship. Is poor communication the problem between Jorge and Marisa? What other problems may be evident in this relationship? Did Marisa make the right choice in this situation? Why?

4.   Alan and Nadia are becoming increasingly intimate. Nadia knows Alan wants to have sex, but she would rather wait until they are married for moral reasons — yet she loves him and doesn't want to seem like a prude. What should she do? Could sex ruin their relationship? What are the benefits of waiting?

Chapter Activities

A.   **Personal Assessment:**
Am I developing healthy sexual relationships? To find out, circle the answer that best applies to you.

		Never		Sometimes		Always
1.	I am comfortable with my gender and sex role.	1	2	3	4	5
2.	I have the ability to form positive interpersonal relationships.	1	2	3	4	5
3.	I have the ability to respond to erotic stimulation with pleasure.	1	2	3	4	5
4.	I have the ability to make mature judgments about sexuality.	1	2	3	4	5
5.	I am comfortable with my sexual orientation.	1	2	3	4	5
6.	I am comfortable communicating about sex with others of my gender.	1	2	3	4	5
7.	I am comfortable communicating about sex with others of opposite gender.	1	2	3	4	5
8.	I am free of sexual dysfunctions.	1	2	3	4	5
9.	I know where to obtain accurate information about sexual relationships.	1	2	3	4	5
10.	I know how to access services about sexual relationships.	1	2	3	4	5

Conclusion:
1.   Add up your score. The maximum score is 50. The higher the score, the higher your ability to develop healthy sexual relationships.

2.   Which area(s) did you score the highest (4 or 5 points)?_____
_____

3.   Which area(s) did you score the lowest (1 or 2 points)?_____
_____

4.   What is one change I could make to increase my ability to develop healthy sexual relationships?

_____

_____

B.   Health Enhancement:

1.   Generate a list of 10 qualities you deem important in a relationship. Can you rank them? Compare your list with other classmates.
2.   Write five questions you would ask if you were a contestant on the TV program "The Dating Game."
3.   Write a real or fictitious "Dear Abby" letter about a relationship. Exchange letters and write a response. Return letters to the original author.
4.   Develop a relationship monitoring grid. Watch several TV sitcoms. Using your grid, record the relationship actions you observe. Critique the TV sitcoms based on your data.

C.   Health Promotion:

1.   List three ways you could be involved in helping to improve the healthy relationships in the general population.
2.   List three ways cultural, environmental (physical or social-economic), political, religious, or health care attitudes/actions could be directly or indirectly involved in improving healthy relationships in the general population.
3.   Suggest one way that you personally could be a "healthy relationship" advocate for each of the two target groups: (1) family; (2) friends.

Chapter Review Test

Multiple Choice: Directions: In the space at the left, write the letter of the choice that best completes each of the following statements:

_____   1. Gender identity refers to an individual's: (p. 407)
    a. reproductive organs
    b. sex role behavior
    c. sexual orientation
    d. intimacy level

_____   2. Sexual orientation refers to: (p. 412)
    a. a person's attraction to individuals of a particular gender
    b. a state of comfort with one's gender and sex role
    c. an ability to respond to erotic stimulation with pleasure
    d. an ability to make mature judgments about sexuality

_____   3. The form of sexual behavior when vaginal intercourse is avoided is called: (p. 413)
    a. sexual abstinence
    b. fellatio
    c. foreplay
    d. coitus

_____   4. According to Robert Sternberg which of the following is NOT a key ingredient of love? (p. 415)
    a. intimacy
    b. passion
    c. infatuation
    d. commitment

_____   5. According to the "Triangular Theory of Love", which type of relationship includes all three components of love? (p. 415)
    a. consummate love
    b. romantic love
    c. fatuous love
    d. compassionate love

_____   6. The biological urge or appetite for sexual activity is also known as: (p. 418)
    a. sexual orientation
    b. libido
    c. sex role identity
    d. intimacy level

_____   7. The erogenous zones include the: (p. 418)
   a. genital and breasts
   b. genitals only
   c. brain and body's extremities like the hands and feet
   d. body's senses, which include smell, taste, and feeling

_____   8. Coitus is another name for: (p. 418)
   a. fellatio
   b. intercourse
   c. entercourse
   d. foreplay

_____   9. The pooling of blood in the genital tissue during sexual excitement is referred to as: (p. 419)
   a. myotonic
   b. orgasm
   c. vasocongestion
   d. resolution

_____ 10. Which of the following conditions generally occurs in both sexes during the plateau phase of the sexual response cycle? (p. 421)
   a. a sex flush
   b. orgasm
   c. vaginal lubrication
   d. impotence

_____ 11. This dysfunction is defined as a persistent or recurrent absence of sexual fantasies and/or a desire for sexual activity. (p. 422)
   a. inhibited sexual desire
   b. erectile dysfunction
   c. impotence
   d. dyspareunia

_____ 12. The inability to achieve and maintain an erection long enough to participate in sexual intercourse is called: (p.423)
   a. impotence
   b. erectile dysfunction
   c. premature ejaculation
   d. dyspareunia

_____ 13. The inability to achieve orgasm by a woman is called: (p. 424)
   a. female orgasmic disorder
   b. vaginisms
   c. impotence
   d. dyspareunia

_____   14. Dyspareunia is a term associated with: (p. 424)
   a.   failure to reach orgasm
   b.   involuntary constriction of the vagina
   c.   painful intercourse
   d.   sexual addiction

_____   15. This therapeutic technique involves learning how to communicate sexual feelings using the nonverbal communication of touch. (p. 424)
   a.   rational motive therapy
   b.   sensate focus therapy
   c.   aversion therapy
   d.   psychotherapy

CHAPTER 16 PRIMER
YOUR SEXUAL BODY: A PRIMER ON REPRODUCTIVE ANATOMY AND PHYSIOLOGY

Chapter Overview

This special primer examines sex and sexuality from an anatomical and physiological perspective so that you can better understand the biological functions of the male and female reproductive systems. The *reproductive system* is a collective term for the tissue and organs responsible for the production of egg or sperm cells and the secretion of sex hormones.

Reproductive Anatomy and Physiology of the Male. One of the primary male reproductive functions is to produce sex cells called *sperm*. The male reproductive system is designed to facilitate the movement of sperm from the sites of production (the testicle) and storage (the epididymis and vas deferens) into the vagina of a female to allow possible union of sperm and egg. Sperm are deposited through a process called *ejaculation*, the expulsion of semen, including sperm, that usually takes place at the peak of sexual excitement, or *organism*.

A second function of the male reproductive system is to produce *androgens*, a family of masculinizing hormones. A third male reproductive function relates to sexual response.

The *scrotum* is a muscular sac located between the penis and the rectum. It forms a pouch for holding the testicles. Sperm are produced in the testicles at a temperature that is three to five degrees below normal body temperature.

Inside each oval-shaped testicle are number *seminiferous tubules* where sperm develop. Surrounding the seminiferous tubules are the *interstitial cells*, the site of hormone production. They are by far the most important source of hormones, particularly testosterone. Sperm produced in the seminiferous tubules migrate to the *epididymis*, where they reside for the two to four weeks it takes to reach maturity. The epididymis also plays a major role in the ability of the sperm to move once they have been ejaculated.

Reproductive Anatomy and Physiology of the Female. The female reproductive system is designed to carry out several functions, including the production of egg cells, the production of hormones, and the gestation and delivery of a baby.

The primary reproductive function of the *ovaries* is to produce egg cells, called *ova*. The production of the hormones estrogen and progesterone is an especially important function of the ovaries. These hormones account for many female characteristics as well as contribute to the success of pregnancy.

The *vagina* is a tubular opening leading to the *cervix*, where sperm must be deposited if pregnancy is to occur. The *fallopian tubes* provide a place for fertilization and the *uterus* provides a location for fetal development as well as the musculature necessary to expel a full-term baby. Finally, like the male, the female genitalia play a primary role in sexual responsiveness.

The *ovary* is the primary sex gland that produces eggs and sex hormones including estrogen, progesterone, and androgens. At birth, a baby girl possesses all the potential egg cells, called *follicles*, necessary for her to remain fertile through a normal period of fertility. Many follicles will begin the maturation process each month, but only one (on rare occasions two or more) will become fully mature as an egg and be released into the abdominal cavity to begin the migration to join the sperm. The release of an egg from the ovary is called *ovulation*.

The Menstrual Cycle. The process of preparing the female body for pregnancy occurs in a cyclic manner beginning at *menarche*, the first sign of menstrual flow, and ending with *menopause*, when fertility and regular menstruation cease. Approximately every month, in response to hormonal signals, the uterus develops the capability of supporting a pregnancy. If pregnancy occurs, the uterus provides a location for fetal development over a nine-month period of gestation. If pregnancy does not occur, the uterus discharges the tissue and fluid build up in preparation for sustaining a pregnancy and begins again the process of preparing for possible pregnancy. This discharge of tissue and fluid is called *menstruation*.

Primer Focus Questions

1.   What anatomical parts make up the <u>external</u> genitalia of the <u>male</u> reproductive system and what are their function?

2.   What anatomical parts make up the <u>internal</u> genitalia of the <u>male</u> reproductive system and what are their function?

3.   In what way is temperature control of the testicles important for fertility in the male?

4.   What route through the male reproductive system do sperm travel starting in the testicles and ending in the penis?

5.   What anatomical parts make up the <u>external</u> genitalia of the <u>female</u> reproductive system and what are their function?

6.   What anatomical parts make up the <u>internal</u> genitalia of the <u>female</u> reproductive system and what are their function?

7.   What female hormones are produced? How would you contrast these with the male hormones and their site of production?

8.   What are follicles and how are they important to the normal fertility period of a female?

9.   What is the difference between "menarche" and "menopause?"

10.   How would you differentiate between the three stages of menstruation?

Primer Review Test

Multiple Choice: Directions: In the space at the left, write the letter of the choice that best completes each
of the following statements.

_____ 1. The muscular sac which forms a pouch for holding the testicles is known as the: (p. 430)
   a. urethra
   b. vas deferens
   c. scrotum
   d. epididymis

_____ 2. The organs of a man's body responsible for the production of both sperm and male hormones
are the: (p. 431)
   a. testes
   b. vas deferens
   c. epididymis
   d. seminiferous tubules

_____ 3. Sperm production takes place within the: (p. 431)
   a. testes
   b. vas deferens
   c. epididymis
   d. seminiferous tubules

_____ 4. The coiled organ that houses maturing sperm cells between two to four weeks is the: (p. 432)
   a. seminal vesicle
   b. vas deferens
   c. epididymis
   d. seminiferous tubules

_____ 5. These two pea-like glands secrete bicarbonate buffers and mucous for lubricating the urethra. (p.
433)
   a. prostate gland
   b. Cowper's gland
   c. seminal vesicle
   d. epididymis

_____ 6. Eggs, or ova, and sex hormones are produced in the: (p. 433)
   a. vagina
   b. fallopian tubes
   c. ovaries
   d. uterus

_____ 7. The most sexually sensitive part of the external reproductive organs in the female body is the (p. 434)
   a. labia majora
   b. labia minora
   c. clitoris
   d. hymen

_____ 8. The release of an egg from the ovary is called: (p. 435)
   a. follicles
   b. fimbriae
   c. menstruation
   d. ovulation

_____ 9. In the female, this muscular organ is also called the womb: (p. 436)
   a. ovaries
   b. uterus
   c. cervix
   d. vagina

_____ 10. The first sign of menstrual flow is referred to as: (p. 436)
   a. menarche
   b. menopause
   c. menstruation
   d. ovulation

_____ 11. When fertility and regular menstruation cease, it is known as: (p. 436)
   a. menarche
   b. menopause
   c. menstruation
   d. ovulation

_____ 12. The number of phases in the menstrual cycle is: (pp. 436-437)
   a. one
   b. two
   c. three
   d. four

_____ 13. The hormone responsible for stimulating the ovary to begin the process of preparing egg cells for ovulation is: (p. 436)
   a. FSH
   b. LH
   c. estrogen
   d. progesterone

_____ 14. The sharp rise in the concentration of this hormone triggers ovulation. (p. 437)
    a. FSH
    b. LH
    c. estrogen
    d. progesterone

_____ 15. This hormone is critical to the maintenance of pregnancy. (p. 433)
    a. FSH
    b. LH
    c. estrogen
    d. progesterone

CHAPTER 17
PLANNING A FAMILY

Chapter Overview

Many choices and options are involved when adults decide whether or not they wish to become parents. This chapter explains the processes and difficulties of conception, pregnancy, and birth and examines various methods of birth control.

The Beginnings of a Family. There are many types of families from the *nuclear family* which includes two parents and their children; the *extended family* of grandparents, cousins, etc.; *dual-career families*, both adults working outside the home; to the *single-parent family*, typically with the mother as the single parent; as well as many other family units such as unmarried couples living together and homosexual partnerships with children.

Marriage and Family. Marriage often includes the decision to have children. One choice towards creating a family involves both partners desiring a child, with both partners physically and psychologically mature as well as financially secure to raise a child. *Infertility*, the inability to conceive, is often due to age, poor health, low sperm count, pelvic infections and stress. Adoption, *artificial insemination, in vitro-fertilization,* hormone therapy, various surgeries, and surrogate motherhood are options for people experiencing conception difficulties. *Preconception care,* involves a *risk assessment* of potential health problems for the mother. Two additional levels of care include: (1) *health promotion* which give parents instructions on how to begin a healthy pregnancy; and (2) *intervention* strategies which are prevention steps designed to be taken before a child is conceived.

A Healthy Pregnancy. One sign that a woman is pregnant is *amenorrhea*, a missed menstrual period. However, a urine test confirming the presence of the hormone, *human chorionic gonadotropin,* is the best indicator. Complete prenatal care helps to insure that the pregnancy will be safe and healthy for both mother and child. Another important aspect of prenatal care involves healthy behaviors on the part of the mother; including not smoking, not drinking alcohol, using caution with all drugs, good nutrition, and exercise. Diagnostic tests to check the development of the fetus are (1) sonograms, (2) blood tests to determine high levels of AFP, (3) an *amniocentesis,* and (4) *a chronic villus sampling* (CVS). All of the above tests are used to detect abnormalities and other characteristics of the fetus. Trimesters, of 13 weeks each, are divisions used to explain different developmental stages of the fetus which occur during a normal pregnancy.

Preparing for Childbirth. Many mothers are opting now to deliver their child in a birthing center, attended by a certified *midwife*, yet there are still many hospital births, especially for those considered high risk. The first stage of labor begins when the cervix, the opening to the uterus, first *effaces*, or thins, and then *dilates* to an opening of roughly 10 cm, the point where the baby's head is seen, called *crowning*. The birth of the baby occurs during the second stage of labor when the uterine contractions are intensified enough to move the baby through the birth canal. Often a physician will perform an *episiotomy*, a cut to widen the vaginal opening. This procedure is considered by many practitioners as unnecessary. One fourth of all births in the United States are delivered by way of a *cesarean section*, a procedure used to remove the baby through an incision in the mother's abdominal wall. This procedure is the choice preferred by most doctors when a child is *breeched* (arriving feet first), or the birth is deemed too risky to be delivered

159

vaginally. The final stage of labor is the expulsion of the *placenta*, the organ attached to the baby by the umbilical cord.

Family Planning is an organized effort for sexual partners to decide if, when, and how to have children, often with the aid of education and contraceptives.

Birth Control: Assuming Responsibility. Contraceptives are methods used to prevent conception that include varying degrees of effectiveness, cost, convenience and safety. Two nontechnological methods are the *rhythm method* which clocks a woman's ovulation cycle, and *withdrawal* of the penis before ejaculation. Hormone contraceptives that keep the woman's body from releasing eggs include the *Pill*, the injection of the drug, *Depo-Provera* and the surgical implant, *Norplant*. Barrier methods include both a male and female *condom*, a soft rubber cup called a *diaphragm* that covers the cervix, and *spermacides* that come in gels, creams, foams and suppositories, for use inside the vagina. Surgical sterilization, a permanent contraceptive technique is referred to as a *vasectomy* in men and *tubal ligation* in women. Another method, the *morning-after pill*, can be used up to 72 hours after unprotected sex.

Abortion Controversy. An *abortion* is terminating a pregnancy. Ninety percent of abortions are performed within the first trimester of a pregnancy by *vacuum aspiration*. This procedure removes the fetus by a suction method. Another abortion procedure is the drug, RU-486, which induces a miscarriage, and is effective 49-63 days after conception. Abortion is a political hotbed in the United States as *pro-life* advocates who wish to see abortion illegal, continually debate with *pro-choice* proponents over abortion legislation.

There are four **Critical Thinking Questions** discussed in this chapter. These questions focus on the supposition that social problems are due to: (1) changing family structures; (2) the ethics of prenatal diagnostic tests when used to determine the sex of the fetus; (3) how to encourage more young adults to use contraceptives as a combination method against unwanted pregnancy and disease; and (4) the reasons for the high rates of unintended pregnancies in the United States.

Chapter Focus Questions

1. What role does the traditional marriage play in the following family structures: nuclear family, extended family and dual-career family?

2. What conditions should a couple consider when choosing whether or not to have children?

3. What factors are believed to be associated with infertility as well as the medical and social efforts to address them?

4. What is the supportive evidence suggesting that preconceptive care and prenatal care are important factors in the health of a pregnancy?

5. What are two methods of studying fetal cells for testing the presence or absence of genetic abnormalities?

6. How would you describe fetal development beginning with conception and carrying through each trimester to birth?

7. How would you describe the process of labor and delivery?

8. In family planning what methods of birth control are chosen by men and which ones by women?

9. What are the characteristics of women who have abortions and what are the reasons they give for choosing to have an abortion?

10. For what reason is family planning most effective when based on high quality information?

Case Study Reflections

In the introduction to chapter 17, Indira and Arjun illustrate successful family planning that culminates in Indira's pregnancy. Louise and Sam illustrate the opposite, as Louise's pregnancy comes before the couple is prepared and after Louise has been drinking and doing drugs.

1.   Identify and explain the dangers for Louise's child as a consequence of her drinking and drug use. How important are the first weeks of gestation?

2.   What steps should Louise and Sam take to insure a healthy development for their child over the remainder of the pregnancy?

3.   How might Louise and Sam respond emotionally to this "surprise" pregnancy? Why might their response be different from that of Indira and Arjun's?

4.   The respective child of each couple may start life in significantly different environments. Compare and contrast the beginning of Indira and Arjun's child experiences with that of Louise and Sam's child. Does this illustrate the importance of family planning? How?

Chapter Activities

A.   **Personal Assessment:**
Am I able to plan a family? To find out, circle the answer that best applies to you.

		Never		Sometimes		Always
1.	My sexual partner and I have similar attitudes about wanting children.	1	2	3	4	5
2.	I am physically healthy enough to raise and care for a child.	1	2	3	4	5
3.	My sexual partner is healthy enough to raise and care for a child.	1	2	3	4	5
4.	I am psychologically healthy enough to raise and care for a child.	1	2	3	4	5
5.	My sexual partner is psychologically healthy enough to care for a child.	1	2	3	4	5
6.	I am mature enough to raise and care for a child.	1	2	3	4	5
7.	My sexual partner is mature enough to raise and care for a child.	1	2	3	4	5
8.	I can provide the necessary economic support the child will need to be healthy and properly nourished.	1	2	3	4	5
9.	My sexual partner can provide the necessary economic support the child will need to be healthy and properly nourished.	1	2	3	4	5
10.	My sexual partner and I have similar attitudes about artificial insemination.	1	2	3	4	5
11.	My sexual partner and I have similar attitudes about in vitro fertilization.	1	2	3	4	5
12.	My sexual partner and I have similar attitudes about surrogate motherhood.	1	2	3	4	5

		Never		Sometimes		Always
13.	I know safety, effectiveness, cost, availability, and convenience information about several contraceptive methods.	1	2	3	4	5
14.	My sexual partner and I have similar attitudes about abortion.	1	2	3	4	5
15.	I know how to obtain reliable information, products, and services related to family planning.	1	2	3	4	5

Conclusion:

1. Add up your score. The maximum score is 75. The higher the score, the higher your readiness for family planning.

2. Which area(s) did you score the highest (4 or 5 points)?_____
_____

3. Which area(s) did you score the lowest (1 or 2 points)?_____
_____

4. What is one change I could make to increase my understanding of, and readiness for, family planning?_____
_____

B.   Health Enhancement:

1. Using the Self-Assessment, survey several individuals of varying ages. Analyze the responses and draw conclusions.
2. What are the pros and cons of a college marriage?
3. Write five guidelines a couple should follow when attempting to resolve a "family planning" conflict.
4. Determine age benchmarks (e.g. 0-5, 6-15, 16-18, 19-22) and the cost of raising a child for each benchmark.
5. A couple wants three children. How should they be spaced? Justify your answer.

C.   Health Promotion:

1. List three ways you could be involved in helping to improve the family planning skills in the general population.
2. List three ways cultural, environmental (physical or social-economic), political, religious, or health care attitudes/actions could be directly or indirectly involved in improving the family planning skills in the general population.
3. Suggest one way that you personally could be a "family planning skills" advocate for each of the two target groups: (1) family; (2) friends.

Chapter Review Test

Multiple Choice: Directions: In the space at the left, write the letter of the choice that best completes each of the following statements:

_____   1.   The type of family that includes those who are connected by blood, marriage or adoption but who live in another location is referred to as a(n): (pp. 442-443)
a. nuclear family
b. extended family
c. dysfunctional family
d. single-parent family

_____   2.   Approximately what percentage of marriages end in divorce in the U.S.? (p. 444)
a. 20%
b. 50%
c. 70%
d. 80%

_____   3.   Most people who divorce: (p. 444)
a. do not remarry
b. eventually remarry
c. move back with their parents
d. move in with their grown children

_____   4.   Infertility is generally defined as the: (p. 448)
a. ability of a couple to conceive twice within a nine month period
b. ability of a couple to conceive once every month
c. inability of a couple to conceive after one year of intercourse without contraception
d. inability of a couple to conceive until they use contraception

_____   5.   A technique in which a women is artificially impregnated by sperm from an unknown donor or sperm from her partner is called: (p. 448)
a. fallopius fertilization
b. artificial uterectomy
c. in vitro fertilization
d. artificial insemination

_____   6.   Which term literally means "fertilization in a glass"? (p. 448)
a. artificial insemination
b. natural insemination
c. in vitro fertilization
d. fallopius fertilization

_____   7. Amenorrhea is: (p. 450)
        a. painful menstruation
        b. premenstrual syndrome
        c. missed menstrual period
        d. delayed menopause

_____   8. What hormone can accurately detect pregnancy about 10 days following conception? (p. 450)
        a. estrogen
        b. progesterone
        c. human chorionic gonadotropin
        d. thalidomide

_____   9. Which of the following maternal behaviors is associated with higher infant mortality and low birth weight babies? (pp. 450-451)
        a. smoking
        b. caffeine consumption
        c. too little exercise
        d. poor hygiene

_____   10. Crowning refers to: (p. 455)
        a. breaking of waters
        b. breech births
        c. when the baby's head is first seen at the vaginal opening
        d. postpartum birth

_____   11. The diagnostic tool that allows the physician indirectly to see the developing fetus and its individual organ systems is called a (an) (p. 452)
        a. chorionic villus sampling
        b. mammogram
        c. cat-scan
        d. sonogram

_____   12. A test of the mother's blood, to evaluate the health of the fetus, can detect levels of this substance produced by the fetus' kidneys. (p. 452)
        a. alpha-fetaprotein
        b. beta-fetaprotein
        c. amniocentesis
        d. thalidomide

_____   13. Both amniocentesis and chorionic villi sampling involve which of the following risks to the mother and fetus? (p. 452-453)
        a. spontaneous abortion
        b. infection
        c. missing or underdeveloped appendages
        d. all of the above

_____   14. A cesarean delivery is: (p. 457)
  a. a breech delivery
  b. delivery without medication
  c. natural childbirth
  d. surgical removal of the baby

_____   15. Depo-Provera is an example of a: (p. 461)
  a. male condom
  b. birth control pill
  c. spermicide
  d. diaphragm

CHAPTER 18
AGING: GROWING OLDER, KEEPING HEALTHY

Chapter Overview

All people age: yet how they age depends on heredity, culture, attitude and health habits. This chapter provides information on what to expect from the aging process and how to make the transition into older age the healthiest and most informed.

Growing Older. *Gerontologists* study the different aspects of aging and measure age by three criteria, *chronological age, functional age, and psychological age.* Prejudices and stereotypes about the elderly, termed *ageism,* usually suggest that most older people are helpless, sick and unable to learn new concepts. Statistics, however, show that most elderly individuals live on their own; are a very diverse group; and most consider themselves quite healthy. Because women tend to live longer than men, more elderly people are female, while elderly men are more likely to be married than women. Why people age differently is due to their style of aging. For example, people have a continuity of habits and personality in their lives that carries over into maturity. Some continue to remain active as they age. Others seem to gradually detach themselves from social ties. Another way to define the process of aging is by depicting it as a series of tasks that need to be completed and are based upon certain psychological stages within a life. Other cultures, as represented in the article about the Japanese, seem to show more respect towards the elderly and make greater efforts than Americans to ease their elders into old age. However, a recent Gallop poll shows that many Americans wish to be more involved in assisting their parents as they age.

Aging Body and Mind: Changes that Occur Over Time. General wear and tear of the body aggravates illnesses for the elderly as they experience a weakened immune system, decreased energy, and organs working less efficiently than when they were younger. Signs of aging include the development of wrinkles, balding and graying of hair, hearing loss for some, accumulation of fat, weakened muscles and the thinning of bones, called *osteoporosis.* Many elderly people experience vision problems such as *presbyopia,* or shortsightedness and *cataracts.* Although, an individual's sex life may change as they age, sexual satisfaction is maintained by many older adults. Long-term memory loss does not occur very often to the elderly, but the time it takes to retrieve knowledge may take longer and the elderly often experience short-term memory loss as their aging brains produce less *neurotransmitters*, necessary for relaying information. The illness that most commonly affects memory and produces *dementia* in the elderly is *Alzheimer's disease,* a degenerative and presently incurable disease.

Preventable Health Problems. One obvious health problem that can be prevented for the elderly is over medication. This health issue often disguises and confounds the real physical or mental health problem. The elderly are at high risk for depression, adverse reactions to drugs as a result of medication abuse, and unintentional injuries, such as falls.

Promoting Healthy Aging. Older adults who eat nutritiously and exercise regularly, even if the exercise is moderate, like walking or Tai chi, will experience better health and a superior quality of life. Since 1982, Americans over the age of 65 have been improving their ability to remain active and independent and are less likely to experience a disability from a chronic disease than in the past.

There are four **Critical Thinking Questions** interjected throughout the chapter. These questions discuss: (1) why in the last ten years there appears to be no increase in the healthy amount of years an elderly person can expect; (2) the theory that aging is a process of disengaging oneself from societal commitments; (3) the connections that are made between physical fitness and independence for the elderly; and (4) how older people's perception of time influences how they make decisions about their health.

Chapter Focus Questions

1. What are the differences between chronological, functional and psychological methods of measuring age?

2. How would you describe the "typical" elderly person according to gender, marital status, living arrangements, and health status?

3. What are some of the misconceptions about aging including the misperception that older people are not sexually active?

4. How would you describe the different "styles" of aging?

5. How does aging influence one's health status?

6. What happens to the bones, the senses and the brain during the aging process?

7. What are some of the myths associated with Alzheimers?

8. How does your brain change with the aging process?

9. How might one go about preventing some of the major health concerns of aging including depression, medicine abuse and accidental falls?

10. How important is regular physical activity and nutritious diet as they relate to healthy aging?

Case Study Reflections

Sam McNeil and Charles Hill are taking two typical but opposite approaches to retirement. Sam is selling his auto repair shop and plans on taking it easy — retiring. Charles plans for "retirement" meanwhile, are much different. His include touring the country and volunteering in his community.

1.   Sam and Charles are presumably the same age chronologically. Compare their years in terms of "functional age" and "psychological age." Who is younger "functionally?" Why? Who is younger "psychologically?" Explain why.

2.   Sam McNeil is one of your grandparents. What would you say to him about his retirement plan? How might you encourage him to stay active?

3.   After only a few months of Sam's retirement, he shows signs of aging. His joints are more stiff, his memory fails frequently, even his hearing seems to be worsening. What is happening to Sam physiologically? Why does it seem to be happening so quickly?

4.   Charles returns after his three-month tour as happy as ever. Sam turns increasingly somber. Explain the psychological differences in the two men. How might Sam deal with his depression?

Chapter Activities

A.   Personal Assessment:

Am I keeping healthy as I grow older? To find out, circle the answer that best applies to you.

		Never		Sometimes		Always
1.	I believe I am healthier than others my chronological age.	1	2	3	4	5
2.	My functional age is lower than my chronological age.	1	2	3	4	5
3.	I will continue to exercise my body as I grow older.	1	2	3	4	5
4.	I will continue to exercise my mind as I grow older.	1	2	3	4	5
5.	I have a "healthy" genetic background.	1	2	3	4	5
6.	I get regular eye examinations.	1	2	3	4	5
7.	I protect my eyes against sun damage.	1	2	3	4	5
8.	I eat a variety of foods.	1	2	3	4	5
9.	I know how to obtain reliable health/aging-related information, products, and services.	1	2	3	4	5

Conclusion:

1.   Add up your score. The maximum score is 45. The higher the score, the greater the likelihood you will stay healthy as you grow older.

2.   Which area(s) did you score the highest (4 or 5 points)?_____

_____

3.   Which area(s) did you score the lowest (1 or 2 points)?_____

_____

4.   What is one change I could make to improve my likelihood of growing older healthy?_____

_____

B.   Health Enhancement:

1.   Design a brochure for senior citizens promoting physical activity.
2.   Develop the tool and survey several senior citizens regarding their physical activity. Summarize your findings.
3.   Complete this statement: "You know you're old when. . ."
4.   Research the percentage of senior citizens in your community. How is it changing?
5.   Create a bumper sticker encouraging a healthy lifestyle in the "growing-older" years.

C.   Health Promotion:

1.   List three ways you could be involved in helping older adults in the general population remain healthy.
2.   List three ways cultural, environmental (physical or social-economic), political, religious, or health care attitudes, actions could be directly or indirectly involved in helping older adults in the general population remain healthy.
3.   Suggest one way that you personally could be a "healthier older adult" advocate for each of the two target groups: (1) family; (2) friends.

Chapter Review Test

Multiple Choice: Directions: In the space at the left, write the letter of the choice that best completes each of the following statements:

_____   1. Specialists who study the social, biological, behavioral, and psychological aspects of aging are called: (p. 477)
a. orthopedics
b. podiatrists
c. gerontologists
d. chiropractors

_____   2. Which biological theory of aging suggests that foreign elements in the blood accumulate over time in the body? (p. 478)
a. wear and tear theory
b. free radicals theory
c. biological clock theory
d. high-density lipoprotein theory

_____   3. Which of the following is NOT considered a common measure of one's age? (p. 478)
a. chronological age
b. functional age
c. psychological age
d. social aging

_____   4. All of the following demographics concerning the elderly are true EXCEPT: (p. 478)
a. The elderly live independently in their own home.
b. There are more elderly women than men.
c. There are less married elderly women than married elderly men.
d. The majority of elderly live in a nursing home.

_____   5. Which of the following statements is NOT true regarding the process of aging? (p. 479)
a. Short-term memory loss does occur.
b. Intellectual judgment and clarity of thinking is impaired.
c. The elderly can assimilate as much overall knowledge as younger people.
d. Sexual activity decreases mostly due to a lack of a partner.

_____   6. This style of aging suggests that both society and the elderly slowly withdraw from each other? (p. 482)
a. disengagement style
b. activity style
c. continuity style
d. disassociation style

_____ 7. The style of aging suggesting that people do not change very much as they grow older is the: (p. 480)
  a. disengagement style
  b. continuity style
  c. activity style
  d. disassociation style

_____ 8. For a grandmother to see her children and grandchildren become adults is a joy, but to watch her great-grandchildren grow up being the ultimate happiness represents a: (p. 482)
  a. sense of identity
  b. sense of trust
  c. sense of generativity
  d. sense of personal integrity

_____ 9. Which of the following is NOT a true statement about aging? (pp. 485-490)
  a. appearance changes
  b. negative attitudes are adopted
  c. bodily functions deteriorate
  d. susceptibility to injuries increases

_____ 10. More people over age 65 die of this chronic health problem than of any other cause. (p. 485)
  a. heart disease
  b. cancer
  c. chronic respiratory ailment
  d. stroke

_____ 11. These organs are among the most resistant to change due to aging provided they are cared for. (p. 485)
  a. heart
  b. lungs
  c. kidneys
  d. liver and pancreas

_____ 12. Which of the following statements is NOT true concerning osteoporosis? (p. 487)
  a. After menopause women are at a significantly decreased risk.
  b. Heredity plays a role in osteoporosis.
  c. The condition is linked to increased calcium loss.
  d. It develops less frequently in men.

_____ 13. Reducing the risk for osteoporosis for women focuses on: (p. 488)
  a. use of hormone replacement therapy
  b. adequate calcium intake
  c. avoiding cigarette smoking and heavy alcohol consumption
  d. all of the above

_____   14. What is a common early symptom of Alzheimer's disease? (p. 490)
a.   inability to write or speak coherently
b.   inability to find the right word
c.   do not understand when people speak to them
d.   may not recognize themselves in the mirror

_____   15. The most common psychological disorder among older people is: (p. 495)
a.   psychosis
b.   neurosis
c.   depression
d.   incontinence

CHAPTER 19
DEATH AND DYING

Chapter Overview

Inevitability for all people, death and dying is often a difficult and painful process. This chapter examines the various perspectives of when, how and why death occurs, the process of dying, and how people deal with the event of death.

Meaning of Death. To understand and explain the expiration of life, many different perspectives have been formulated. From a biological viewpoint, death may occur when cardiovascular and respiratory functions cease, or when brain activity is no longer apparent. Brain activity, by the way, is measured by an *electroencephalogram* (EEG). Many religious perspectives see death as the moment the soul has left the body. These definitions often become controversial when examined from a legal perspective, especially in right-to-die cases. For example, while *physician-assisted suicide* is considered illegal, other forms of euthanasia are legal. Yet people have wide and differing opinions on what is a dignified death. *Passive euthanasia* is the withholding of food or fluids to a dying person, while *active euthanasia* is an action taken to hasten death, i.e. lethal injections. Individuals can create a *living will* or *advance medical directive* that specifies the type of medial treatment they would want if they became terminally ill. A *durable power of attorney for health care* may be appointed who is responsible to carry out the patient's requests. Examples of these types of documents are included in the chapter. Age determines how a person will react to and comprehend death. While children usually see death as reversible or preventable, young adults often see themselves as invincible. On the other hand, the older a person becomes, the less likely they are to participate in risky behavior and become more philosophical about death.

Dying as a Process. The time between when it is apparent that a person will die of a known cause and the actual state of death is called the *living-dying interval*. The psychiatrist, Elizabeth Kuebler-Ross, identified five stages of death many people experience when told of a terminally ill condition. These include *denial, anger, bargaining, depression,* and *acceptance*. Throughout all these stages, the patient always displays some expression of hope. Hospice programs, whether conducted at inpatient treatment centers or within a patient's home, were developed to give a dying person and their loved ones comfort and support within a framework of health care.

For Survivors: A Time of Decisions and Bereavement. When someone has died, decisions regarding disposal of the body must be made. People today are able to make funeral arrangements before they die, to insure that their wishes are met and remove the burden from loved ones of having to make decisions during a time of grief. Many people have signed a uniform donor card, indicating they would like their organs donated. Sometimes the body is *embalmed* in preparation for an open casket funeral. Other times the body is burned in a process call *cremation*, and the ashes are scattered or kept in a family urn. The urn then is usually kept either at home or placed in a *columbarium* at a cemetery. Most cultures honor the dead with some sort of ceremony. Depending on the family, there may be more than one ceremony involved. For example, a funeral may be accompanied by a Catholic wake or Jewish shiva. During the *bereavement* period of *mourning,* someone may go through various stages of grief beginning with the *impact* of the news that a loved one has died, a period of *recoil* or trying to behave normally, and finally *recovery*.

There are three **Critical Thinking Questions** within the chapter. The first question examines the lack of public health policy dealing with issues of death, primarily creating dignified deaths. The second examines what forces determine a society's acceptance of ordained deaths. The third question discusses the legality of euthanasia as an involuntary decision on the part of the patient.

Chapter Focus Questions

1. How is death biologically, legally and religiously understood?

2. Why is euthanasia considered so controversial in our society?

3. How is death as it is perceived by children different than the way it is understood by adolescents and adults?

4. How is the process of dying differentiated from the living-dying interval?

5. How does Elizabeth Kubler-Ross, describe the stages of dying?

6. In what ways does a hospice function to provide comfort for dying patients?

7. What tasks should survivors undertake in the event of a loved one's death?

8. How does a living will differ from a durable power of attorney for health care?

9. How would you describe the three stages of grieving?

10. How might grief lead to an inspiration or recommitment to life?

Case Study Reflections

In the introduction to chapter 19, George and Krista are both diagnosed with terminal illnesses. George refuses to acknowledge his approaching death and dies without preparation and with much pain. Krista recognizes the extent of her illness. She talks it over with her family and makes arrangements to die in her own home.

1.   George refuses to acknowledge all five stages of the dying process. Which ones does he experience? How does his refusal to acknowledge several of these stages make him more bitter about his impending death?

2.   How may being young affect the way George and Krista deal with their own death? How might the recent death of a loved one help them cope with their own timely death?

3.   "Hope is crucial for coping with dying." Through the lives of George and Krista, how is this statement verified? What happens when hope fades?

4.   Krista spends time talking with her brother about her impending death. After reading the chapter on death, do you think it helped her in preparing for her death? How did it help the family? Contrast this situation with George's family.

Chapter Activities

A.   Personal Assessment:

What are my attitudes toward death and dying? To find out, circle the answers that best applies to you.

		Never		Sometimes		Always
1.	I support passive euthanasia.	1	2	3	4	5
2.	I support active euthanasia.	1	2	3	4	5
3.	I support physician-assisted suicide.	1	2	3	4	5
4.	I will have (or do have) a living will.	1	2	3	4	5
5.	I support and favor cremation.	1	2	3	4	5
6.	I support and favor embalming.	1	2	3	4	5
7.	I support open casket reviewal.	1	2	3	4	5
8.	I support donor cards.	1	2	3	4	5

Conclusion:

1.   Add up your score. The maximum score is 40. The higher, or lower, the score, the greater you adhere to your attitudes, beliefs and values about death and dying.

2.   Which area(s) did you score the highest (4 or 5 points)?_____
_____

3.   Which area(s) did you score the lowest (1 or 2 points)?_____
_____

4.   What is one change I could make to improve my understanding of issues related to death and dying?_____
_____

B.   Health Enhancement:

1.   Using Dr. Elisabeth Kubler-Ross' work on the emotional stages of grieving or dying individuals as a foundation, write a brief case study on someone you know.
2.   Should a funeral be planned before or after death? Justify your answer?
3.   Compare the dying and death customs in varying cultures around the world.
4.   Write several guidelines to follow when speaking to a grieving individual.

5.   Find and write down five inspirational quotes you would find comforting in a time of death or dying. Share your list with classmates.

C.   Health Promotion:

1.   List three ways you could be involved in helping the general population better understand death and dying issues.
2.   List three ways cultural, environmental (physical or social-economic), political, religious, or health care attitudes/actions could be directly or indirectly involved in improving death and dying issues in the general population.
3.   Suggest one way that you personally could create better understanding of death and dying for each of the two target groups: (1) family; (2) friends.

Chapter Review Test

Multiple Choice: Directions: In the space at the left, write the letter of the choice that best completes each of the following statements:

_____ 1. The biological definition of death involves: (p. 506)
- a. irreversible loss of all body functions
- b. the cessation of cardiac and respiratory activity
- c. the cessation of heartbeat and breathing
- d. all of the above

_____ 2. When a person no longer has brain activity but breathing is controlled by a respirator, the individual is said to be: (p. 506)
- a. legally dead
- b. brain dead
- c. comatose
- d. functionally dead

_____ 3. Brain death is confirmed by a(n): (p. 506)
- a. sonogram
- b. electroencephalogram
- c. brain scan
- d. electrocardiogram

_____ 4. A person in a vegetative state is: (p. 507)
- a. completely unresponsive
- b. able to remove own bodily wastes
- c. able to eat on his/her own
- d. aware of his/her environment

_____ 5. This type of euthanasia is exemplified when a patient is allowed to bring about his/her own death through a lethal injection or other means provided by the physician. (p. 508)
- a. assisted suicide
- b. passive euthanasia
- c. clinical death
- d. medical suicide

_____ 6. The removal of a feeding tube from a dying or comatose patient is an example of: (p. 508)
- a. assisted suicide
- b. passive euthanasia
- c. active euthanasia
- d. medical suicide

_____ 7. Withholding something needed to maintain life, such as not putting a dying person on a respirator is: (p. 508)
    a. assisted suicide
    b. passive euthanasia
    c. active euthanasia
    d. clinical death

_____ 8. A legal document stating that a terminally ill person desires to die peacefully and with dignity is referred to as a: (p. 511)
    a. legal will
    b. living will
    c. dying will
    d. donor card

_____ 9. A durable power of attorney for health care: (p. 511)
    a. Is a representative from the legal rank who speaks for your health care whether you are able to or not.
    b. Must be a lawyer who makes decisions for your health-care if you are unable to do so.
    c. Must be a health/medical professional who makes decisions for your health care.
    d. May be any person who is aware of your wishes and can speak for your health care if and when you are unable.

_____ 10. Which of the following is a true statement about a 5 year old's conceptual awareness of death? (p. 512)
    a. death is a normal part of life
    b. death is blamed on an external force such as a "bogeyman"
    c. deny that death is final
    d. the dead go to an underworld

_____ 11. The dying process begins with a diagnosis of a terminal disease or condition and continues until the point of death; a period called: (p. 514)
    a. the bereavement period
    b. the living-dying interval
    c. the grieving period
    d. the beginning period

_____ 12. Which of the following emotional stages of dying does the terminal patient refuse to believe that he or she is going to die? (p. 515)
    a. denial
    b. anger
    c. bargaining
    d. depression

_____   13. This specialized health care program emphasizes the management of pain and other symptoms associated with terminal illness. (p. 515)
   a.   health maintenance programs
   b.   drug therapy
   c.   hospice care
   d.   none of the above

_____   14. Which of the following is a document stipulating which parts of the body may be used in the event of death? (p. 519)
   a.   living will
   b.   will
   c.   donor card
   d.   dying will

_____   15. The process of preserving a body using chemicals for open casket viewing is called: (p. 520)
   a.   cremation
   b.   columberium
   c.   embalming
   d.   entombment

CHAPTER 20
LIVING IN A HEALTHY ENVIRONMENT

Chapter Overview

Much of the earth and its resources are damaged or in the process of being contaminated by various pollutants. This chapter explains environmental hazards found in the air, water, and food supply and teaches the individual how to reduce and help prevent contamination.

Environmental Health: How Big is the Problem? An *acceptable risk* is a theory that certain environmental problems pose too little harm to cause much concern. However, many scientists believe that this is a dangerous approach to analyzing environmental hazards, primarily because *multiple hazards* compound themselves and people's reactions to pollutants vary. Pollutants which are *carcinogens* cause cancer, while *teratogens* are responsible for some birth defects. *Mutagens* create changed body cells that are genetically transferred to following generations.

The Air You Breathe. There are many substances in the air that cause irritation as well as more serious health problems to people who inhale the toxins. Asthma is one of the most common health problems associated with air pollution, but other pollutants are known to aggravate and/or cause various cancers and other diseases. The principal air pollutants are: (1) *carbon monoxide*, emitted from motor vehicles; (2) *sulfur oxides*, found in industrial fuels and the cause of *acid rain;* (3) *hydrocarbons*, the primary source being gasoline; (4) *particulates* such as soot or coal dust; (5) *lead;* and (6) *nitrogen oxides* which form *ozone*. The combined result of all these air pollutants in our atmosphere causes a greenhouse effect, which may eventually lead to a *global warming* of the earth.

The Water You Drink. Pollutants in drinking water come from industries, agricultural chemicals, and municipal sources such as leaking septic systems. *Point source pollutants* originate from a particular site while *nonpoint pollutants* contaminate water by means of runoff or seepage. Pollutants such as soils, herbicides, pesticides and toxic waste not only pollute drinking water, but affect living organisms on the food chain, eventually leading to human consumption.

Solid Waste: The Art of Throwing Things Away. To reduce the amount of solid waste that is dumped into landfills, two efforts of conservation are (1) *precycling*, whereby the consumer makes a conscious effort not to purchase products that will contribute to excessive waste; and (2) *recycling* which is the collection and reuse of many types of solid waste.

Health Hazards from Toxic Waste. When *toxic chemicals* are incorrectly disposed of in landfills or toxic waste dumps, they can cause toxic poisoning to exposed persons through contaminated water, breast milk and food.

Dangers from Noise. Noise over 85 decibels can cause damage to the cilia in your inner ear, also known as the *cochlea*. Short term hearing loss caused from a single loud noise is called a *temporary threshold shift*. Repeated exposure to loud noises, however, may cause permanent hearing loss.

Indoor Pollution: Sick Buildings, Sick People. People afflicted by *tight building syndrome*, a condition caused by superior insulation of buildings, experience dizziness, nausea, and other irritations due to breathing unhealthy air. Other indoor pollutants are carbon monoxide and nitrogen dioxide from wood and coal stoves; and radon. Proper ventilation, correct storage of chemicals, air purifiers and repairing old heaters can all help reduce indoor air pollution.

Environmental Ethics. Opinions about the environment range from aggressive anti-environmentalism, whose proponents believe that nature should be utilized completely for human consumption, to radical environmentalism, whose supporters actively campaign to protect all living things from dangerous human encroachments. Most people take a middle ground approach, believing that caution should be taken with the earth's resources to protect it for future generations.

There are four **Critical Thinking Questions** within the chapter. They include: (1) the difficulties in measuring environmental hazards; (2) the concerns with adding fluoride to a community's drinking water; (3) who should control the economics of recycling; and (4) how privacy issues may conflict with public policies to regulate public health concerns.

Chapter Focus Questions

1.   How do serious environmental threats differ from threats that are perceived to be serious, but actually present little risk to the global environment?

2.   Why is it difficult to measure environmental health threats?

3.   How might you define carcinogen, teratogen and mutagen?

4.   What are the health effects of air pollution?

5.   What are the principle water pollutants and their source in the environment?

6.   What are the health threats of solid waste?

7.   What practices of precycling and recycling are used in an effort towards reducing solid waste?

8.   What are the health hazards of toxic wastes in the environment?

9.   How is noise an environmental pollutant?

10.   What is the range of opinion concerning environmental policy and action?

Case Study Reflections

At the beginning of chapter 20, Angela and Karim take a long hike in nature. Angela doesn't understand or respect nature. As an example, she develops diarrhea from drinking the stream water. She also clutters the environment by leaving a plastic bag on the trail. Karim, on the other hand, respects nature by avoiding the unhealthy water and not polluting the environment.

1.   What is the source of Angela's disregard for nature? How do you contrast that from Karim's? How does this translate into the way the two experience and treat nature?

2.   What does Angela's experience with polluted water tell us about "pristine" nature? From the chapter, describe the extent of pollution in the environment.

3.   "It's just one plastic bag," Angela says later about her littering. What's the problem with this line of thinking?

4.   "Karim's a freak about nature," Angela says of him. Analyze Karim's environmental awareness. Is he too radical? Why or why not? Is it socially acceptable to be environmentally conscious? Explain.

Chapter Activities

A.   Personal Assessment:

Am I living in a healthy environment? To find out, circle the answer that best applies to you.

		Never		Sometimes		Always
1.	Air pollution can cause serious ill health effects.	5	4	3	2	1
2.	The outside air that I breathe is healthy.	5	4	3	2	1
3.	The inside air that I breathe is healthy.	5	4	3	2	1
4.	I am exposed to passive smoking.	1	2	3	4	5
5.	I am exposed to carbon monoxide.	1	2	3	4	5
6.	I am exposed to sulfur oxides.	1	2	3	4	5
7.	I am exposed to nitrogen oxides.	1	2	3	4	5
8.	I am exposed to ozone poisoning.	1	2	3	4	5
9.	I am exposed to smog.	1	2	3	4	5
10.	I am exposed to unsafe drinking water.	1	2	3	4	5
11.	I recycle.	5	4	3	2	1
12.	I am exposed to hazardous (toxic) wastes.	1	2	3	4	5
13.	I am exposed to hazardous noise levels.	1	2	3	4	5
14.	I have high environmental ethics.	5	4	3	2	1
15.	I know how to file an environmental complaint.	5	4	3	2	1
16.	I know how to obtain reliable environmental-related information, products, and services.	5	4	3	2	1

Conclusion:

1.   Add up your score. The maximum score is 80. The higher the score, the higher your environmental health risk.

2.   Which area(s) did you score the highest (4 or 5 points)?_____

_____

3.   Which area(s) did you score the lowest (1 or 2 points)?_____

_____

4.   What is one change I could make to improve the health in my environment?_____

_____

B.   Health Enhancement:

1.   Invent a product, or product concept, that would improve environmental health.
2.   Design a T-shirt that promotes an environmental health issue.
3.   Write a mini-mystery based on an environmental health issue.
4.   Using the Personal Assessment, survey several individuals of varying age. Summarize and report your findings.
5.   Make up five riddles focusing on improved environmental health. Share with classmates.

C.   Health Promotion:

1.   List three ways you could be involved in helping to improve the health environment in the general population.
2.   List three ways cultural, environmental (physical or social-economic), political, religious, or health care attitudes/actions could be directly or indirectly involved in improving the health environment in the general population.
3.   Suggest one way that you personally could be a "health environment" advocate for each of the two target groups: (1) family; (2) friends.

Chapter Review Test

Multiple Choice: Directions: In the space at the left, write the letter of the choice that best completes each of the following statements:

_____   1. The type of toxic chemical capable of promoting birth defects is referred to as being: (p. 530)
  a. carcinogenic
  b. pharmogenic
  c. mutagenic
  d. teratogenic

_____   2. When a substance is capable of promoting genetic alterations in cells, it is said to be: (p. 530)
  a. carcinogenic
  b. pharmogenic
  c. mutagenic
  d. teratogenic

_____   3. Today, the single most significant cause of air pollution is: (p. 530)
  a. the automobile
  b. industrial toxins
  c. natural sources
  d. manufacturing corporations

_____   4. Benzene is a dangerous gaseous pollutant to humans because of its ability to cause: (p. 531)
  a. cancer
  b. heart disease
  c. stroke
  d. liver disease

_____   5. This colorless, odorless and poisonous gas that originates primarily from motor vehicle emissions is: (p. 532)
  a. carbon monoxide
  b. carbon dioxide
  c. carbon oxide
  d. bicarbonate

_____   6. The primary origin of sulfur oxides is: (p. 532)
  a. motor vehicle emissions
  b. electrical utilities and industrial plants
  c. household chimneys
  d. dumping of hazardous wastes

_____ 7. The type of air pollution caused by the combination of sulfur oxides and particulate matter is: (p. 532)
   a. ozone
   b. smog
   c. acid rain
   d. greenhouse effect

_____ 8. A substance produced primarily by coal plants and industrial processes associated with causing black lung and brown lung diseases is: (p. 533)
   a. asbestos
   b. lead
   c. sulfur oxide
   d. particulates

_____ 9. A poisonous form of oxygen that is produced when nitrogen dioxide reacts with hydrogen chloride is: (p. 533)
   a. nitrogen oxide
   b. hydrocarbons
   c. ozone
   d. chlorofluorocarbons

_____ 10. The ozone layer: (p. 534)
   a. is a colorless, odorless, poisonous gas
   b. is formed from sulfur oxides
   c. filters out ultraviolet rays from the sun
   d. is formed by high levels of nitrogen oxide

_____ 11. Global warming that results from solar heat being trapped by air pollutants is known as: (p. 535)
   a. particulate pollution
   b. ozone pollution
   c. hydrocarbon pollution
   d. the greenhouse effect

_____ 12. Chloroflurocarbons, chemicals that contribute to the depletion of the ozone layer, are found in: (p. 534)
   a. aerosol spray propellants
   b. lead products
   c. industrial boilers
   d. electric power plants

_____ 13. What chemical is added to drinking water to prevent outbreaks of cholera and dysentery? (p. 536)
   a. fluoride
   b. chlorine
   c. phosphates
   d. nitrates

_____ 14. This source of water pollution may include urban storm water runoff, bacteria from leaking septic systems, and water table contamination from landfill seepage. (p. 538)
   a. industrial
   b. municipal
   c. agricultural
   d. household

_____ 15. All BUT which of the following are sensible ways to reduce the amount of solid waste in the environment. (pp. 541-543)
   a. precycle
   b. recycling trash
   c. reducing the amount of product packaging
   d. using more disposable products

CHAPTER 21
MAKING HEALTH CARE DECISIONS

Chapter Overview

Because Americans spend more on health care than citizens of any other country, the choices regarding insurers, medication, physicians, and other medical services are often of an economic nature and require informed decision making on the part of the consumer. This chapter: (1) details various health care options, (2) explains the dispensation of medications, and (3) teaches the reader how to be wary of health care fraud.

Buying Health Care: How Do Consumers Make Decisions? The best way for individuals to take responsibility for their own health is to obtain accurate and unbiased information from health care reference books, periodicals, professional web pages (useful listings found in the chapter), or by reading the FDA's *patient package inserts* before purchasing health care products. Advertisements can use misleading or vague information to promote products by: (1) claiming scientific research, (2) promoting its popularity with the *bandwagon approach* ("everyone is buying it"), (3) using *testimonials* of people asserting its success, (4) appearing to sentiment with *emotional appeals* of the product's trustworthiness, and (5) with providing a *price appeal* by a *comparison to other products*. Quack medicine, often quoted as 'quick cures' and 'medical breakthroughs,' defraud people, who are ill-informed about scientific health care, of their money. Consumers should recognize that they need to ask for information, exercise caution, choose products wisely, and issue complaints when services or medications do not live up to their claims or cause physical damage.

How to Choose Health Care Providers. In addition to medical doctors, there are various other licensed health care practitioners and alternative health care professionals, such as *Naturopaths,* who combine various types of treatment methods based on an individual's specific needs. Medical facilities include: (1) *primary care* or *outpatient care* in a physician's office or in the emergency room, (2) *secondary care* or *inpatient care* which takes place in a community hospital, and (3) tertiary care, found at a hospital that specializes in a certain type of procedure.

Paying for Health Care. Although most health care is provided through insurance companies and paid for by employers, schools, or the individual, many people in this country are *uninsured* or *underinsured.* What this means is, they are unable to pay costs not covered by their insurance plans. Or in another way, they may receive inadequate medical coverage from their particular insurer. Health insurance policies vary, so it is important to be familiar with common terms (listed in the chapter) and to be informed about different types of coverage.

The *indemnity plan* is a *fee-for-service* insurance provider where patients would pay their own medical costs, and then be reimbursed. Another kind of insurance is the Managed Care Plans. These plans are of three different types: (1) *health maintenance organizations* or HMOs, where all health care is directed by a single physician or internist; (2) *point-of-service plans,* where patients can see practitioners outside the plan for an additional fee; and (3) *preferred provider organizations* where the patient may choose a physician from a group in order to receive a discounted copayment.

Drugs as Medicine. About one half of all prescription drugs are misused, usually because the patient failed to ask for, follow, or read instructions. Questions individuals should ask their physician or pharmacist before taking any medication are: (1) the name and purpose of the medication, (2) the possible side effects, (3) substances and activities to avoid while taking the medication, (4) when and how to take it, and (5) if there is any additional written information about the medication. When seeking information about medication, try to compare sources, use data from well-known organizations and be ready to distrust any source that can not be backed up by another source.

There are four **Critical Thinking Questions** within the chapter. They include: (1) the trustworthiness of health care product information sources; (2) the necessary criteria for reporting adverse drug reactions to the FDA; (3) the ethics of refusing emergency medical treatment to the uninsured; and (4) the benefits gained when prescriptions are accompanied by written and/or verbal information.

Chapter Focus Questions

1.   What is the role of information in consumer decision making?

2.   What advertising techniques are used to promote health products and services?

3.   Is there a difference between quackery and health fraud?

4.   What are one's rights as a consumer of health-related products and services?

5.   How does one file a consumer complaint when dissatisfied with a product?

6.   What strategies make for a wise decision when selecting a physician?

7.   What are the differences between the insured, the uninsured and the underinsured?

8.   What are the advantages and disadvantages of traditional indemnity plans, health maintenance organizations and preferred provider organizations?

9.   What are the differences between prescription and over-the-counter drugs?

10.   How are hotlines and the Internet considered sources of health information?

Case Study Reflections

Chapter 21 begins with Rani purchasing the miracle tummy reducer that promises to take "inches from her mid-section," but fails to reduce anything. George is also overweight, but he develops a sound diet and a weekly exercise program that produces visible results.

1.   What advertising techniques did Rani respond to? To what consumer weakness does the tummy reducer speak?

2.   Do you think the miracle tummy reducer might have worked if Rani had used it over a longer period of time? Why are so many people "taken in" by such gizmos?

3.   What is the difference between Rani's approach to making healthy decisions and George's approach? What considerations does Rani need to keep in mind when making choices about a health product?

4.   What is the principle behind George's health style that makes him successful in achieving his health goals?

Chapter Activities

A.   **Personal Assessment:**

Am I able to make good health care decisions? To find out, circle the answer that best applies to you.

		Never		Sometimes		Always
1.	I am actively involved in my own health care decisions.	1	2	3	4	5
2.	I have complete information concerning my health.	1	2	3	4	5
3.	I understand all of the tests that physicians and other health care workers perform on you.	1	2	3	4	5
4.	I understand the variables associated with the purchase of prescription drugs.	1	2	3	4	5
5.	I understand the variables associated with the purchase of over-the-counter (OTC) drugs.	1	2	3	4	5
6.	I have the information and knowledge to make reliable and unbiased health care choices.	1	2	3	4	5
7.	I am able to analyze health care advertising.	1	2	3	4	5
8.	I know how to file a health care consumer complaint.	1	2	3	4	5
9.	I know how to choose a health care provider.	1	2	3	4	5
10.	I know how to choose health insurance.	1	2	3	4	5
11.	I know how to obtain reliable health care-related information, products, and services.	1	2	3	4	5

Conclusion:

1.   Add up your score. The maximum score is 55. The higher the score, the more "health care" literate you are.

2.   Which area(s) did you score the highest (4 or 5 points)?_____
_____

3.   Which area(s) did you score the lowest (1 or 2 points)?_____
_____

4.   What is one change I could make to improve my health care literacy?_____

_____

B.   Health Enhancement

1.   Create a game that matches health care specialists with their field of expertise. (e.g. Oncologist — cancer).
2.   List the pros and cons of choosing a doctor in a group practice over a doctor in private practice.
3.   Research the types and availability of health care plans and insurance available for varying individuals (e.g. young, old, employed, unemployed).
4.   List several important guidelines to consider when selecting a health care facility.
5.   Create a cartoon about health care insurance and/or facilities.

C.   Health Promotion:

1.   List three ways you could be involved in helping to improve the understanding of health care decisions in the general population.
2.   List three ways cultural, environmental (physical or social-economic), political, religious, or health care attitudes/actions could be directly or indirectly involved in improving the health care decisions in the general population.
3.   Suggest one way that you personally could create better understanding of the health care decisions for each of the two target groups: (1) family; (2) friends.

Chapter Review Test

Multiple Choice: Directions: In the space at the left, write the letter of the choice that best completes each of the following statements:

_____   1. The primary purpose of advertising is to: (p. 561)
   a. provide accurate information
   b. assist customers in making wise choices
   c. provide an understanding of the nature of health fraud
   d. sell products or services

_____   2. This advertising appeal to the consumer makes use of celebrities who inform consumers of how well the product worked for them. (p. 562)
   a. emotional appeal
   b. testimonials
   c. bandwagon approach
   d. scientific studies

_____   3. Using this appeal, advertisers sell a product by claiming that "everyone is using the product." (p. 562)
   a. emotional appeal
   b. testimonials
   c. bandwagon approach
   d. scientific studies

_____   4. A health claim made by a product or service that cannot be justified by scientific evidence is called: (p. 562)
   a. hi-jacking
   b. homeopathy
   c. quackery
   d. truth-telling

_____   5. Which forms of illnesses are most commonly prone to quackery treatments: (p. 562)
   a. cancer and arthritis
   b. skin disorders
   c. kidney and liver diseases
   d. psychosomatic illnesses

_____   6. Which of the following is considered a patient's right regarding health care products and services? (pp. 563-564)
   a. receive considerate and respectful care
   b. turn down all medical treatment
   c. see all hospital records
   d. refuse payment if the treatment is unsuccessful

_____ 7. Which of the following offices regulates unfair and deceptive advertising? (p. 564)
   a. Better Business Bureau
   b. Consumer Product Safety Commission
   c. Federal Trade Commission
   d. Food and Drug Administration

_____ 8. This alternative form of treatment is based on the healing power of nature and so uses such methods as acupuncture and herbal medicine. (p. 565)
   a. osteopathy
   b. chiropractic medicine
   c. podiatry
   d. naturopathy

_____ 9. Medical care provided in hospitals specializing in open-heart surgery and organ transplants would be an example of: (p. 569)
   a. primary care
   b. secondary care
   c. inpatient care
   d. tertiary care

_____ 10. The federal program which provides health care for those 65 years of age or older is: (p. 569)
   a. Medicaid
   b. Medicare
   c. disability insurance
   d. HMO group practice

_____ 11. The established amount of money that the insuree must pay before the insurer will reimburse for services is called the: (p. 571)
   a. coinsurance
   b. copayment
   c. deductible
   d. pre-existing conditions

_____ 12. This traditional method of obtaining health insurance coverage allows you to pay for most of your medical bills and then file a claim to be reimbursed is: (p. 571)
   a. cost-sharing
   b. fee-for-service
   c. copayment
   d. deductible

_____   13. The type of managed care plan that assigns you to a family physician or internist who acts as the gatekeeper to all other health services provided by the organization is: (p. 573)

a.   prepaid group practice (PGP)

b.   health maintenance organization (HMO)

c.   point-of-service plan (POS)

d.   preferred provider organization (PPO)

_____   14. One advantage HMO's have over other managed health care plans is that HMO's: (pp. 573-574)

a.   tend to offer one-step shopping

b.   offer more services

c.   copayment is lower

d.   offer patients a wider choice of physicians

_____   15. Drugs ordered specifically by the physician since they are considered unsafe for use except under professional supervision are called: (p. 575)

a.   over-the-counter drugs

b.   prescription drugs

c.   brand name drugs

d.   generic drugs

ANSWERS TO CHAPTER PRACTICE TESTS

Chapter 1: Multiple Choice Items

1. C (p.4)	6. B (p.8)	11. A (p.13)
2. D (p.4-5)	7. B (p.10)	12. A (p.13)
3. A (p.5-6)	8. B (p.11)	13. D (p.14)
4. D (p.7)	9. A (p.10)	14. B (p.14)
5. A (p. 6)	10. B (p.11)	15. C (p.15)

Chapter 2: Multiple Choice Items

1. B (p.25)	6. A (p.27)	11. B (p.34)
2. B (p.25)	7. C (p.28)	12. A (p.35)
3. A (p.26)	8. B (p.29)	13. C (p.35)
4. C (p.27)	9. B (p.32)	14. A (p.35)
5. D (p.27)	10. A (p.32)	15. B (p.37)

Chapter 3: Multiple Choice Items

1. B (p.49)	6. B (p.51)	11. B (p.57)
2. A (p.49)	7. C (p.52)	12. D (p.57)
3. D (p.50)	8. D (p.54)	13. C (p.63)
4. D (p.49)	9. C (p.54)	14. B (p.64)
5. B (p.51)	10. A (pp.54-55)	15. B (pp.65-66)

Chapter 4: Multiple Choice Items

1. D (p.75)	6. C (p.77)	11. A (p.85)
2. C (p.75)	7. A (pp. 78-79)	12. B (p.86)
3. B (p.77)	8. C (p.79)	13. C (p.88)
4. D (p.77)	9. B (p.78)	14. B (p.90)
5. D (p.77)	10. D (p.81)	15. D (p.90)

Chapter 5: Multiple Choice Items

1. D (p.97)	6. D (p.98)	11. C (p.100)
2. A (p.97)	7. C (p.100)	12. A (p.101)
3. A (p.97)	8. A (p.100)	13. D (p.102)
4. B (p.97)	9. D (p.100)	14. C (p.104)
5. A (p.98)	10. B (p.100)	15. A (p.107)

Chapter 6: Multiple Choice Items

1. B (p.127)	6. C (p.131)	11. D (p.135)
2. D (p.127)	7. B (p.131)	12. B (p.139)
3. D (p.128)	8. C (p.131)	13. A (p.139)
4. A (p.128)	9. D (p.131)	14. A (p.140)
5. D (p.129)	10. C (p.135)	15. B (p.141)

Chapter 7: Multiple Choice Items

1. D (pp.155-156)	6. B (p.163)	11. D (p.165)
2. B (p.158)	7. D (p.163)	12. A (p.165)
3. C (p.160)	8. C (p.163)	13. A (p.166)
4. D (pp.160-161)	9. D (p.165)	14. D (p.167)
5. A (p.163)	10. B (p.165)	15. D (pp. 167-168)

Chapter 8: Multiple Choice Items

1. D (p.181)	6. B (p.185)	11. B (p.190)
2. A (p.181)	7. C (p.185)	12. D (p.190)
3. A (p.183)	8. A (p.185)	13. A (p.190)
4. B (p.183)	9. D (p. 186)	14. A (pp.190-191)
5. A (p.183)	10. B (p.186)	15. B (p.193)

Chapter 9: Multiple Choice Items

1. B. (p.207)	6. A (p.213)	11. C (p.215)
2. D (p.208)	7. B (p.213)	12. B (p.218)
3. A (p.209)	8. B (p.214)	13. D (p.218)
4. D (p.210)	9. A (p.214)	14. D (p.218)
5. C (p.212)	10. C (p.207)	15. B (p.226)

Chapter 10: Multiple Choice Items

1. C (p.233)	6. B (p.240)	11. B (pp.242-243)
2. B (p.236)	7. C (p.241)	12. D (p.243)
3. B (p.237)	8. B (p.241)	13. C (p.243)
4. C (p.238)	9. C (pp.241-242)	14. D (p.244)
5. D (p.240)	10. B (p.242)	15. B (p.244)

Chapter 11: Multiple Choice Items

1. D (p.265)	6. D (p.269)	11. D (p.276)
2. D (pp.266-267)	7. D (p.273)	12. B (p.276)
3. C (p.267)	8. B (p.273)	13. B (p.277)
4. A (p.269)	9. B (p.274)	14. A (p.278)
5. B (p.269)	10. D (p.274)	15. C (p.283)

Chapter 12: Multiple Choice Items

1. C (p.290)	6. B (p.292)	11 C (p.296)
2. C (p.291)	7. A (p.292)	12. B (p.296)
3. D (pp.292-293)	8. D (p.292)	13. B (p.300)
4. A (p.291)	9. C (p.293)	14. C (p.302)
5. C (p.292)	10. D (p.293)	15. D (p.304)

Chapter 13: Multiple Choice Items

1. D (p.317)	6. C (p.322)	11. A (p.326)
2. D (p.317)	7. C (p.323)	12. B (p.326)
3. B (p.318)	8. A (p.324)	13. A (p.332)
4. A (p.319)	9. B (p.325)	14. A (p.334)
5. D (p.319)	10. C (p.325)	15. D (p.338)

Chapter 14: Multiple Choice Items

1. A (p.353)	6. D (pp.357-358)	11. B (p363)
2. C (p.355)	7. C (p.358)	12. C (p.370)
3. B (p.355)	8. A (p.359)	13. C (p.371)
4. C (p.355)	9. B (p.359)	14. A (p.371)
5. D (p.358)	10. A (p.362)	15. B. (p.375)

Chapter 15: Multiple Choice Items

1. C (p.383)	6. B (p.389)	11. C (p.393)
2. C (p.381)	7. B (p.390)	12. A (p.393)
3. C (p.386)	8. D (p.391)	13. D (p.394)
4. A (p.387)	9. B (p.392)	14. D (p.394)
5. D (pp.389-390)	10. A (p.392)	15. B (p.399)

Chapter 16: Multiple Choice Items

1. B (p.407)
2. A (p.412)
3. A (p.413)
4. C (p.415)
5. A (p.415)
6. B (p.418)
7. A (p.418)
8. B (p.418)
9. C (p.419)
10. A (p.421)
11. A (p.422)
12. A (p.423)
13. A (p.424)
14. C (p.424)
15. B (p.424)

Chapter 16 Primer: Multiple Choice Items

1. C (p.430)
2. A (p.431)
3. D (p.431)
4. C (p.432)
5. B (p.433)
6. C (p.433)
7. C (p.434)
8. D (p.435)
9. B (p.436)
10. A (p.436)
11. B (p.436)
12. C (pp.436-437)
13. A (p.436)
14. B (p.437)
15. D (p.437)

Chapter 17: Multiple Choice Items

1. B (pp.442-443)
2. B (p.444)
3. B (p.444)
4. C (p.448)
5. D (p.448)
6. C (p.448)
7. C (p.450)
8. C (p.450)
9. A (pp.450-451)
10. C (p.455)
11. D (p.452)
12. A (p.452)
13. D (pp.452-453)
14. D (p.457)
15. B (p.461)

Chapter 18: Multiple Choice Items

1. C (p.477)
2. B (p.478)
3. D (p.478)
4. D (p.478)
5. B (p.479)
6. A (p.482)
7. B (p.480)
8. D (p.482)
9. B (pp.485-490)
10. A (p.485)
11. B (p.485)
12. A (p.487)
13. D (p.488)
14. B (p.490)
15. C (p.495)

Chapter 19: Multiple Choice Items

1. D (p.506)
2. B (p.506)
3. B (p.506)
4. A (p.507)
5. A (p.508)
6. C (p.508)
7. B (p.508)
8. B (p.511)
9. D (p.511)
10. B (p.512)
11. B (p.514)
12. A (p.515)
13. C (p.515)
14. C (p.519)
15. C (p.520)

Chapter 20: Multiple Choice Items

1. D (p.530)	6. B (p.532)	11. D (p.535)
2. C (p.530)	7. B (p.532)	12. A (p.534)
3. A (p.530)	8. D (p.533)	13. B (p.536)
4. A (p.531)	9. C (p.533)	14. B (p.538)
5. A (p.531)	10. C (p.534)	15. D (pp.541-543)

Chapter 21: Multiple Choice Items

1. D (p.561)	6. A (pp.563-564)	11. B (p.571)
2. B (p.562)	7. C (p.564)	12. B (p.571)
3. C (p.562)	8. D (p.565)	13. B (p.573)
4. C (p.562)	9. D (p.569)	14. A (pp.573-574)
5. A (p.562)	10. B (p.569)	15. B (p.575)